Quality Indicators

Defining and Measuring Quality in Psychiatric Care for Adults and Children

Report of the APA Task Force on Quality Indicators
and
Report of the APA Task Force on
Quality Indicators for Children

Quality Indicators

Defining and Measuring Quality in Psychiatric Care for Adults and Children

Report of the APA Task Force on Quality Indicators
and
Report of the APA Task Force on
Quality Indicators for Children

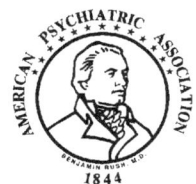

Published by the American Psychiatric Association
Washington, DC

Note: The authors have worked to ensure that all information in this book is accurate at the time of publication and consistent with general psychiatric and medical standards, and that information concerning drug dosages, schedules, and routes of administration is accurate at the time of publication and consistent with standards set by the U.S. Food and Drug Administration and the general medical community. As medical research and practice continue to advance, however, therapeutic standards may change. Moreover, specific situations may require a specific therapeutic response not included in this book. For these reasons and because human and mechanical errors sometimes occur, we recommend that readers follow the advice of physicians directly involved in their care or the care of a member of their family.

The findings, opinions, and conclusions of these reports do not necessarily represent the views of the officers, trustees, all members of the task forces, or all members of the American Psychiatric Association. Task force reports are considered a substantive contribution of the ongoing analysis and evaluation of problems, programs, issues, and practices in a given area of concern.

Manufactured in the United States of America on acid-free paper
05   04   03   02   4   3   2   1
First Edition

American Psychiatric Association
1400 K Street, N.W.
Washington, DC 20005
www.psych.org

Library of Congress Cataloging-in-Publication Data
APA Task Force on Quality Indicators
    Quality indicators : defining and measuring quality in psychiatric care for adults and children : report of the APA Task Force on Quality Indicators and report of the APA Task Force on Quality Indicators for Children.—1st ed.
       p. ; cm.
    Includes bibliographical references and index.
    ISBN 0-89042-291-5 (alk. paper)
    1. Mental health services—Standards. 2. Quality assurance.
    I. APA Task Force on Quality Indicators for Children. II. Title.
    [DNLM: 1. Mental Health Services—standards. 2. Health Services Accessibility—standards. 3. Outcome Assessment (Health Care)—standards. 4. Quality Indicators, Health Care—standards.
WM 30 A10455q 2002]
RA790.5 .A633 2002
362.2'02'18—dc21

                       2002018296

British Library Cataloguing in Publication Data
A CIP record is available from the British Library.

Contents

**Report of the American Psychiatric Association
Task Force on Quality Indicators**

Report of the American Psychiatric Association Task Force on Quality Indicators for Children

Introduction

There was a time, not so long ago, when quality could be defined by saying "I know it when I see it." Not so today. The public is restive. They want to know that the medical care they receive is safe, effective, and accessible to them. Purchasers of care (principally business and government, who together account for over 80% of health care purchases) are moving beyond making cost the overriding variable in what benefits and services are supplied to subscribers. Purchasers want clear, reliable, meaningful, and comparable information on what care is provided and with what results. Medical professionals fervently want the quality dimension restored to health care purchase decisions after more than a decade of intrusive, for-profit management practices in a market-driven economy.

The field of quality measurement in health care, including psychiatric care, while still young, developed remarkably in the past 10 years. Quality can be defined, measured, reported, and compared among clinical facilities and health plans, and data can be used to improve the care that patients and their families receive. At first, quality measurement was a retrospective review of what was done and with what problems. Then accrediting agencies like the Joint Commission on Accreditation of Healthcare Organizations (JCAHO) and the National Committee for Quality Assurance (NCQA) began requiring reports on selected indicators of quality. The government's Health Care Financing Administration (HCFA; now the Centers for Medicare and Medicaid Services, or CMS) also began mandating some federally funded programs to use specified indicators as conditions for payment. The reports by the Institute of Medicine (IOM) on medical errors and on quality, reinforced by great media attention, lent further credibility and impetus to the development of measures that assess health care quality in ways that can be publicly reported. More recently, clinicians and professional societies have joined these forces in a manner that emphasizes clinically meaningful measures of quality.

In 1997, with strong encouragement from Samuel Guze, M.D., then chair of the Council on Research, Rodrigo Muñoz, M.D., president-elect of the American Psychiatric Association (APA), established a task force under the auspices of the APA Council on Quality Improvement in order to develop quality measures for general (principally adult) psychiatric care. John M. Oldham, M.D., was named chair of the APA Task Force on Quality Indicators. The task force was charged with developing clinically based, patient-focused quality indicators that use existing and ongoing research and clinical consensus in selecting potential indicators. The task force also worked closely with the APA Steering Committee on Practice Guidelines to identify existing and future quality indicators that are linked to the evidence base that underlies all APA practice guidelines. The task force issued its report in March 1999, after approval by the APA Board of Trustees.

One of the task force's recommendations was to create the APA Task Force on Quality Indicators for Children to focus exclusively on the special issues related to children and adolescents. The Task Force on Quality Indicators for Children, chaired by James C. MacIntyre II, M.D., began its work in 1999 and received APA Board of Trustees approval of its report in the fall of 2001. Throughout the development of the Report on Quality Indicators for Children, the task force maintained ongoing communication and collaboration with the American Academy of Child and Adolescent Psychiatry.

Both reports sought to offer a clinical framework for quality measurement that would provide sample indicators of quality rather than produce a comprehensive compendium of relevant quality indicators.

This monograph assembles and publishes both these task force reports for the first time. This publication represents an ongoing effort on the part of the APA to lend its professional expertise to the vital activity of defining measures of quality for treatment of adults and children. The focus of these reports, and the measures offered, are at the level of health plans, facilities, and systems of care, not individual clinicians. Both these reports recommend using the indicators to examine quality in clinical practice, to stimulate research, and to foster the development of additional indicators.

The initial task force report (March 1999) focuses primarily on adults, and the more recent task force report (October 2001) focuses on children and adolescents. Each task force report begins with a conceptual framework for clinically based indicators for the treatment of psychiatric and substance use disorders. Measures of the structure of the care delivery system, clinical processes of care provided to patients, and the outcomes of care were carefully explored in the development of each report. The definitions of an indicator, measure, standard, priority area, and dimension of care were carefully developed and used consistently in both reports. A matrix of priority areas of care, including specific populations of patients (e.g., the elderly, seriously and persistently mentally ill, developmentally disabled, and others) and diagnostic categories (e.g., depressive disorders, substance use disorders, schizophrenia, bipolar disorder, personality disorders, and others), was considered by each task force. Important aspects of patient care were examined and a framework was constructed. This quality framework included dimensions (domains) of access, quality (or appropriateness of care), perceptions of care (also known as satisfaction), and outcome. The children's report also included the important area of prevention in the quality framework.

Each report uses the same format consisting of dimensions (domains) of care, recommended goals, indicators, measures, and standards. Sample indicators of quality were formulated for each recommended goal. An *indicator* was defined as an important component of quality patient care. Important principles guided the selection process of indicators. Both task forces sought to develop indicators that were clinically meaningful, could be used to improve patient care, could be quantified in a practical and feasible manner, were evidence based, and had minimal potential for being "gamed." For each indicator, the task forces provided sample measures (a means of quantifying the indicator) and standards (a level of the measure that is suggestive of quality). Because benchmarks for comparative quality standards are still uncommon, the task forces drew on what research and clinical consensus did exist, while appreciating that many standards will need to be changed as these indicators are used in clinical practice. Each task force also carefully considered numerous relevant methodological issues: cultural, linguistic, and ethnic differences; data collection and tracking; confidentiality of data; risk adjustment; use of rating scales and standardized instruments; and designation of standards.

The following are several recommended quality goals from the task force report on general (adult) psychiatric care:

- Patients with serious and persistent mental illness should have access to newer generations of antipsychotic medications as they become available.

- Psychotherapy, psychiatric rehabilitation, and other psychosocial treatments should be used in appropriate intensity and duration for those disorders for which they have been shown to be effective.
- Health care systems or plans should regularly and systematically solicit information from their patients (and their families, when involved in treatment) and from individual clinicians providing care within their organizations about their perceptions and experiences of the care provided.
- Patients receiving treatment known to be effective for their conditions should experience a significant reduction in symptoms/signs after receiving appropriate treatment for a reasonable period of time.

Examples of specific quality indicators from this report include

- Access to new antipsychotics for patients with schizophrenia.
- Appropriate use of psychosocial treatment (like Assertive Community Treatment) for severely and persistently mentally ill patients.
- Assessment by health plans of patients' perception of care.
- Reduction in frequency of panic attacks among patients with the diagnosis of panic disorder in a given health plan.

The following are several recommended quality goals from the Task Force on Quality Indicators for Children:

- The mental health status of children and adolescents should be assessed yearly utilizing a method or measure appropriate for the child's age and development.
- Children and adolescents should have timely access to appropriately qualified clinicians for psychiatric evaluations, other assessments, and treatment.
- Children with severe or persistent mental illness whose care involves multiple child serving systems, caregivers, and service providers should have their care coordinated.
- The level of functioning for children and adolescents receiving treatment known to be effective for their condition(s) should improve after receiving appropriate treatment for a reasonable period of time.

Examples of specific quality indicators from this report include

- Plans provide access to anti–obsessive-compulsive disorder (OCD) medication for child or adolescent patients diagnosed with OCD.

- Adolescents diagnosed with depression, OCD, or other anxiety disorders have a trial of cognitive-behavioral therapy (CBT) of appropriate intensity and duration.
- Adolescent members using mental health or substance abuse services are either very or highly satisfied with their services.
- Reduced use of substances among patients with a diagnosis of a substance-related disorder (abuse or dependence) who are receiving treatment for the disorder in a given health plan.
- Reduction in family's stress level and impact of illness.

Each task force labored to make the reports readable and user-friendly. Both reports principally consist of a section titled "Workbook of Quality Indicators." These respective sections function as a menu of numerous quality indicators that are divided into the different dimensions of care. Readers can select a particular dimension or individual indicators of interest. In addition, the report on child indicators contains a glossary of important terms and their definitions. Both reports contain a listing of acronyms and abbreviations and an index of indicators by topic. Finally, each report has an extensive reference and bibliography section with complete citations for all references in the reports.

The task force chairs and members offer this monograph as an initial step in what must be an ongoing effort by clinicians to define, measure, report, and improve the care that patients and their families receive. Much more work needs to be done. We hope that these reports will be of interest to those who receive our care and to those who provide it, to those who accredit and regulate care, and to those who purchase and administer clinical services. To the extent that we have furthered an early and ongoing journey into quality measurement by clinicians, consumers, and purchasers of health care, we regard our efforts in creating these reports and this monograph as successful.

Lloyd I. Sederer, M.D.
John M. Oldham, M.D.
James C. MacIntyre II, M.D.
November 2001

Report of the American Psychiatric Association Task Force on Quality Indicators

Approved by the APA Board of Trustees March 13, 1999

Task Force on Quality Indicators

Contents

Executive Summary

Charge and Process

In September 1997, the American Psychiatric Association (APA) leadership expressed its view that the association should begin the development of clinically based, patient-focused quality indicators utilizing existing and ongoing research and clinical consensus. As a result, the APA Task Force on Quality Indicators was established under the auspices of the Council on Research and the Council on Economic Affairs, with the strong support of President-Elect Rodrigo Muñoz. Each member of the task force brings a different perspective. Several are APA representatives to accrediting bodies, some with expertise in indicators or accreditation, others in particular systems or populations, and still others in APA's practice guidelines.

As requested, the task force produced a framework for developing clinically based quality indicators and a set of example indicators specific to psychiatric and substance abuse treatment. The framework was based on a matrix of priority areas and dimensions of treatment. Recommendations for each aspect of the framework were also developed. The example indicators, which include measures and standards, correspond with the recommendations. The recommendations, which are directed to health facilities, plans, and systems, address significant concerns in psychiatric and substance abuse treatment. The indicators themselves are exemplars, intended to serve as an initial approach to evaluating mental health care provided by organized systems of care and as a source of direction for additional research and development of new indicators.

In presenting its report, the task force emphasizes that the development of quality indicators is a work in progress. The specific examples of indicators given here are not intended to be comprehensive. Many indicators could be substituted to address other important aspects of the broad recommendations about clinical care. Some of the sample indica-

tors are supported by an extensive empirical evidence base; others have more limited research support. Some are more fully developed than others. The degree of practicality and the expense of collecting data required by the indicators vary considerably and are discussed in the full report. The task force encourages others to examine, challenge, or support with research the examples of indicators it is setting forth. It hopes that others will build on its experience to expand the number of useful indicators in the field of mental health, including substance use disorders.

The task force undertook a thoroughgoing process in developing the recommendations in this report. It reviewed work in progress by other organizations. It established priority concerns and relevant recommendations. It defined terms and principles for selection of indicators. And, it solicited advice from consultants and several APA components. The process is described more completely in the report, as are the principles that guided selection of indicators.

Definitions and Framework

The working definitions used by the task force are

Recommendation/goal: an important clinical principle that reflects quality patient care
Indicator: a component of quality patient care
Measure: a mechanism or instrument to quantify the indicator
Standard: the level of the measure that suggests that the component of care is of adequate quality (When currently available information does not permit specificity, the level of standard may be used on a comparative basis.)

The framework for discussion and selection of possible quality indicators is as follows:

A. **Access**

   1. To effective medication
   2. To effective psychosocial treatment
   3. To appropriate specialized services

B. **Quality**

   1. Comprehensive evaluation
   2. Appropriate use of medication

3. Appropriate provision of psychosocial treatment
4. Appropriate use of screening and prevention services

C. Perceptions of care

1. Patient
2. Family
3. Clinician

D. Outcome

1. Improved level of functioning and quality of life and minimization of social and economic cost
2. Reduction and/or stabilization of symptoms

Recommendations and Selected Indicators

The underlying recommendations are found in Section V of the report of the task force; indicators, measures, standards, and discussion are found in the workbook, Section VI.

Other APA Efforts

This project complements a range of existing APA efforts. For example, in APA's development and updates of practice guidelines, potential quality indicators are identified and operationalized. Another APA project focuses on the development of quality indicators for children and adolescents in health care systems. Diagnosis and assessment projects, such as DSM-IV and the APA *Handbook of Psychiatric Measures,* and other projects such as the report of the Task Force on Electroconvulsive Therapy aim to foster scientifically and clinically appropriate standards. In addition, the APA routinely comments on drafted quality indicators proposed by the government and other quality oversight organizations.

Report Use and Dissemination

The task force believes that its report will be of interest to everyone involved in the mental health services system—those who use and provide services, those who accredit and purchase them, and those who oversee access and delivery. The report will be distributed to appropriate offices and agencies of federal and state government; voluntary accrediting organizations; collegial, medical, and professional associations; consumer advocacy groups; managed care organizations; managed behavioral health organizations; and purchasers. The task force hopes to stimulate dialogue with each of these audiences and to advocate strongly for the delivery of high-quality psychiatric treatment and mental health services, including substance abuse treatment, to all who require them.

Report of the Task Force on Quality Indicators

I. General Context

A. Trends in the Field

Faced with a rapidly changing health care system, consumers and purchasers of health care services in this country increasingly demand quality and value. Patients want assurances that they will receive services that enhance their health. Facilities, practitioners, and health plans strive to upgrade the quality of the care they deliver, while at the same time informing consumers, payers, and accrediting organizations of their progress in maintaining or improving quality. Developing methods for assessing quality of care has thus become a major concern of governmental agencies, professional associations, advocacy groups, health care plans and facilities, and accrediting organizations. Their many initiatives share the goal of defining the elements of quality treatment and designing systems to capture and report that information.

Whether particular quality indicators are actually used by health care plans, organizations, and systems depends on several factors: the data sources available; the cost and burden of collecting, analyzing, and reporting data; and the costs of buying or developing measurement systems. The choice of indicators may also be influenced by the unique mission or population served or by the requirements of accrediting organizations.

B. Initiatives of a Variety of Accrediting Organizations

Recognizing the importance of performance measurement, national accrediting bodies have incorporated quality measures into their evaluations of health care systems, plans, and programs. Among the organizations that have taken a lead are the Joint Commission on

Accreditation of Healthcare Organizations (JCAHO) and the National Committee for Quality Assurance (NCQA). A consumer group, the President's Advisory Commission on Consumer Protection and Quality in the Health Care Industry, has also recognized the importance of assessing quality of performance. As noted in its November 1997 report, the group includes performance measures in information for consumers about health plans and health providers.

The scarcity of widely recognized psychiatric performance measures prompted the NCQA to appoint a Behavioral Health Measurement Advisory Panel to develop quality indicators. For the same reason, JCAHO postponed requiring free-standing psychiatric facilities and systems to select a performance measurement system until March 1999, a year after such systems were required of other health care facilities.

Although many accrediting organizations are integrating performance measurement into their accreditation processes, each focuses on different levels of health care delivery. For example, JCAHO accredits a range of health care facilities, including those that provide acute, ambulatory, behavioral health, home, long-term, and managed care. NCQA focuses on systems of care for defined populations. The American Medical Accreditation Program (AMAP) focuses on physician-specific indicators.

JCAHO, through its "Agenda for Change," is placing increasing importance on continuous quality improvement (CQI). Its ORYX program integrates performance measurement into the accreditation process. The long-range goal of this initiative is "to establish a data-driven, continuous survey and accreditation process to complement the standards-based assessment." Accredited facilities (not including psychiatric facilities) were expected to contract with an ORYX-approved performance measurement system by March 1998 and begin collecting data on a portion of their patient population. Free-standing psychiatric facilities providing 24-hour care were extended a 1-year delay to chose a performance measurement system. Their selection was due on March 1, 1999. Data will be transmitted to JCAHO during 1999 and then used to inform the accreditation process. Data of psychiatric facilities will be transmitted in 2000. JCAHO will continue to raise standards for demonstrating quality by requiring that, each year, accredited facilities must increase the percentage of their patient populations on whom performance measurements are collected.

NCQA assesses and reports on the quality of managed care plans. Its Healthplan Employer Data and Information Set (HEDIS) contains measures intended to meet the information needs of managed care plans, group purchasers, consumers, and other users. NCQA has indicated it intends to integrate HEDIS reporting into its accreditation process. The 2000 version of HEDIS will include six measures pertaining to mental health and chemical dependency. A measurement advisory panel is now working to review the current version of the HEDIS measurement set and identify gaps, recommend key quality indicators via a systematic review, and plan for the implementation, monitoring, and improvement of proposed indicators.

AMAP, an initiative of the American Medical Association, is a voluntary, comprehensive accreditation program that measures and evaluates individual physicians against national standards, criteria, and peer performance in five areas: credentials, personal qualifications, environment of care, clinical performance, and patient care results. The measures of clinical performance and patient care results have not yet been developed.

The **American Accreditation HealthCare Commission** (formerly known as the Utilization Review Accreditation Commission) does not currently integrate performance measurement in its accreditation processes. The organization intends to do so in the future, however.

JCAHO, NCQA, and AMAP Collaboration

JCAHO, NCQA, and AMAP have begun collaborating on an initiative to coordinate performance measurement activities across the entire health care system. A jointly sponsored Performance Measurement Coordinating Council (PMCC) will "work to ensure that measurement driven assessment processes are efficient, consistent, and useful for the many parties that rely on them to help make important decisions about health care."

II. APA Context

The APA has been involved, in a variety of ways, with major health care accrediting organizations as they institutionalize data collection and the use of quality indicators nationwide. Carefully constructed research to determine the most valid and meaningful indicators, the ideal approach, will take several years. In the meantime, the APA has begun developing clinically based, patient-focused quality indicators from existing and ongoing research and clinical consensus.

The APA Task Force on Quality Indicators was established in late 1997 at the recommendation of Samuel B. Guze, M.D., Chair of the APA Council on Research, with support from Lawrence Y. Kline, M.D., Chair of the APA Council on Economic Affairs, and APA President-Elect Rodrigo Muñoz, M.D. Task force members bring different perspectives to the effort. Several are APA representatives to accrediting bodies, whereas others have expertise with indicators or accreditation, particular systems, or APA's practice guidelines.

The task force is chaired by John M. Oldham, M.D. Members include Sara C. Charles, M.D., Helen L. Egger, M.D., Anthony F. Lehman, M.D., Denis J. Milke, M.D., Charles E. Riordan, M.D., and Lloyd I. Sederer, M.D. Corresponding members are Lawrence Y. Kline, M.D., and Samuel B. Guze, M.D. A liaison member from the American Academy of Child and Adolescent Psychiatry is Joseph R. Mawhinney, M.D.

Harold Alan Pincus, M.D., Deborah A. Zarin, M.D., Claudia Hart, and Beatrice Edner are key staff members participating in this APA effort.

III. Task Force Approach

A. Goals of Project

The task force was charged to produce a framework for the development of quality indicators and an initial set of indicators for health facilities, plans, and systems that address significant concerns in psychiatric and substance abuse treatment. The set of indicators is intended to serve as a tool for health care groups, including accrediting organizations; as an approach to evaluate care provided by health plans and organized systems of care; and as a source of direction for additional research and development of new indicators. The work of the task force will lend coordination to the APA's liaison with different accrediting and regulating bodies and may serve as a foundation for new strategic alliances to improve care.

The task force was not expected to produce a comprehensive set of indicators, but rather to focus on major clinical concerns in mental health and substance abuse care. Other important and valid measures will no doubt emerge. The recommendations are broad, and the indicators given are not necessarily comprehensive. Some of the examples are supported by an extensive empirical evidence base and may be more fully specified, whereas others have more limited research support and are less well developed.

B.   Process

In the course of its work, the task force

- Examined types of indicators (e.g., structure, process, outcomes).
- Discussed whose performance is to be evaluated by the indicators advanced by the APA.
- Agreed on definitions of terms, such as *indicator, measure, standard, priority area,* and *dimension.*
- Developed a matrix of priority areas and dimensions of treatment.
- Developed a set of selected recommendations relating to quality of care in these priority areas and dimensions.
- Developed principles and criteria for selection of specific indicators.
- Developed an initial set of quality indicators corresponding to the selected recommendations.
- Completed a standard information form for each indicator under consideration.
- Sought input from APA components regarding the indicators under consideration.
- Consulted with experts in health services research.
- Reviewed selected proposed indicators for consistency with APA practice guidelines.
- Sought support from within APA to advance the selected indicators for use and/or consideration by external accrediting bodies, government agencies, and others.

In the course of its work, the task force developed a standard description for each indicator that included the title and description of the indicator, rationale, definition of measure, numerator and denominator, problems or issues in measurement (including reliability and validity of measures), data quality, potential data sources, potential users and delivery settings, description of the standard, and references. This process facilitated fuller consideration of each proposed indicator.

The APA components whose input was solicited included the Assembly; Joint Reference Committee; Council on Addiction Psychiatry;

Council on Aging; Council on Children, Adolescents and Their Families; Council on Economic Affairs; Council on Psychiatric Services; Council on Research; Committee on Health Services Research; Committee on Standards and Survey Procedures; Steering Committee on Practice Guidelines; and the Commission on Psychotherapy by Psychiatrists.

C. Definitions

The task force agreed on the following definitions:

Recommendation/goal: an important clinical principle that reflects quality patient care
Indicator: a component of quality patient care
Measure: a mechanism or instrument to quantify the indicator
Standard: levels of the measure that suggest that the component of care is of adequate quality (When currently available information does not permit specificity, the level of measure may be used on a comparative basis.)

Indicators address various aspects of care and are frequently seen as applicable to structure, process, or outcomes. Many of the existing indicators address structure; they generally look at whether organizational resources and arrangements are in place to deliver quality health care. Some indicators address process by looking at a series of actions, events, mechanisms, or steps. Outcome indicators, which look at the result of a function or process, make up the smallest number of the three types of existing indicators because they require the most sophisticated data collection. Yet, outcome indicators may provide the most direct assessment about whether quality care is actually being delivered. The task force agreed that a good evaluation program may include all three types, giving emphasis to outcome indicators, where possible.

When research and experience are available, thresholds for particular indicators may be specified for acceptable performance. If research is insufficient to support such benchmarks, indicators may still be used to compare performance. In the process of operationalizing indicators, it is important to designate whether available data make it possible to set thresholds or whether comparisons should instead be made with prior performance or data from similar systems. The many challenges, complexities, and limitations in applying available data to the development of quality indicators are widely recognized (1).

Indicators may measure the performance of an individual provider or of a hospital or a network of providers in a health care plan. Entire systems, such as a state mental health system, may also be examined. So many entities are involved in providing care (often interrelated) that the task force found itself using the term system flexibly. Given its mandate, the task force selected indicators that depend on aggregate data—that is, they measure the performance of plans and systems, not of individual providers.

The task force identified **priority areas** and chose some of them for the development of an initial set of quality indicators:

Population categories

- Children and adolescents
- Elderly
- Seriously and persistently mentally ill
- Developmentally disabled
- Abused women
- Head injured
- HIV-AIDS

Diagnoses

- Depressive disorders
- Substance use disorders
- Dual diagnosis (major mental illness and substance use disorders)
- Schizophrenia
- Bipolar disorder
- Disruptive disorders
- Dementia
- Trauma and posttraumatic stress disorder
- Personality disorders

The task force considered **dimensions** of treatment for each of the priority areas. The most useful dimensions are those that can be defined, measured, and improved. After considerable examination and discussion, the task force decided to give greatest importance to the dimensions of access, quality, perception of care, and outcome.

D. Principles

The task force agreed on the following principles to guide selection of indicators:

- The indicator concerns an important aspect of care.
- The indicator is useful in identifying opportunities for improving care.
- The indicator is practically quantifiable.
- Where possible, the indicator can be documented by evidence-based practice guidelines, such as those developed by the APA.
- The indicator minimizes the potential for "gaming" the measure or for unintended adverse consequences.
- Eventually, as a set of indicators is developed and promoted by the APA, the indicators should achieve a balance across priority areas and dimensions of treatment.

IV. Overall Quality Framework From a Clinical Perspective

Focusing on the priority areas and dimensions noted above, the task force constructed the following **framework** for discussing and selecting possible quality indicators:

A. Access
1. To effective medication
2. To effective psychosocial treatment
3. To appropriate specialized services

B. Quality
1. Comprehensive evaluation
2. Appropriate use of medication
3. Appropriate provision of psychosocial treatment
4. Appropriate use of screening/prevention services

C. Perceptions of care
1. Patient
2. Family
3. Clinician

D. Outcome

1. Improved level of functioning and quality of life and minimization of social and economic cost
2. Reduction and/or stabilization of symptoms

V. Recommendations/Goals and Sample Quality Indicators for Selected Areas of Focused Quality Assessment and Improvement

A. Access

A.1. Access to effective medication

Recommendation/goal A.1.1: Patients with severe and persistent mental illness should have access to newer generations of antipsychotic medications as they become available.

> **Sample indicator A.1.1:** Access to new antipsychotics for patients with schizophrenia

Recommendation/goal A.1.2: Patients with substance dependence should have access to clinically appropriate maintenance medications.

> **Sample indicator A.1.2:** Access to effective maintenance medication for patients with opioid or alcohol dependence

> **Sample indicator A.1.3:** Access to effective maintenance medication for inpatients with nicotine dependence

A.2. Access to effective psychosocial treatment

Recommendation/goal A.2.1: Patients with severe personality disorders should have access to psychotherapy, the intensity and duration of which should be determined by the patient's clinical condition.

> **Sample indicator A.2.1:** Access to psychotherapy for patients with borderline personality disorder

A.3. Access to appropriate specialized services

Recommendation/goal A.3.1: ECT should be an available treatment option.

> **Sample indicator A.3.1:** Availability of ECT for patients for whom it is clinically indicated

Recommendation/goal A.3.2: Children and adolescents should have access to appropriate psychiatric evaluation and treatment services.

> **Sample indicator A.3.2:** Availability of appropriate specialized services for prepubertal children with depression in a given health plan

B.   Quality

B.1.   Comprehensive evaluation

Recommendation/goal B.1.1: Patients with new onset of cognitive impairment need a comprehensive assessment that rules out treatable causes of that impairment.

> **Sample indicator B.1.1:** Assessment of cognitive impairment for individuals with new onset of symptoms

B.2.   Appropriate use of medications

Recommendation/goal B.2.1: Medications should be used in appropriate dosage and duration for those disorders for which they have been shown to be effective.

> **Sample indicator B.2.1:** Current treatment with an antidepressant medication for patients with major depressive disorder, moderate or severe

> **Sample indicator B.2.2:** Current treatment with a mood stabilizer for patients with bipolar I disorder

B.3.   Appropriate use of psychosocial treatments

Recommendation/goal B.3.1: Psychotherapy, psychiatric rehabilitation, and other psychosocial treatments should be used in appropriate intensity and duration for those disorders for which they have been shown to be effective.

> **Sample indicator B.3.1:** Appropriate use of psychosocial treatment for a severely and persistently mentally ill population

B.4.   Appropriate use of screening/prevention services

Recommendation/goal B.4.1: Inquiries should be made about the status and functioning of children of parents with psychiatric disorders associated with significant dysfunction.

Sample indicator B.4.1: Screening of children at risk for psychiatric disorders in a given health plan

Recommendation/goal B.4.2: Patients receiving psychiatric evaluations should be explicitly asked about current substance use and evaluated for the presence and/or history of substance use disorders.

Sample indicator B.4.2: Screening of patients for substance use disorders

C. Perceptions of Care

C.1. *Patient*

Recommendation/goal C.1.1: Health care systems or plans should regularly and systematically solicit information from their patients about their perceptions and experiences of the care provided.

Sample indicator C.1.1: Assessment of patients' perception of care

C.2. *Family*

Recommendation/goal C.2.1: When families are involved in treatment, health care systems or plans should regularly and systematically solicit information from families about their perceptions and experiences of the care provided.

Sample indicator C.2.1: Assessment of families' perception of care

C.3. *Clinician*

Recommendation/goal C.3.1: Health care systems or plans should regularly and systematically solicit information from individual clinicians providing care within their organizations about their perceptions and experiences of the care provided by the organization.

Sample indicator C.3.1: Assessment of clinicians' perceptions of care

D. Outcome

D.1. *Improved level of functioning and quality of life, and minimization of social and economic cost*

Recommendation/goal D.1.1: Many patients with mental illness that significantly impairs functioning should be able to resume some degree of productive occupational or educational activity after receiving treatment known to be effective for their conditions.

> **Sample indicator D.1.1:** Resumption of productive activities by patients with severe and persistent mental illness when no longer in the acute phase of illness

D.2. Reduction and/or stabilization of symptoms/signs

Recommendation/goal D.2.1: Patients receiving treatment known to be effective for their conditions should experience a significant reduction in symptoms/signs after receiving appropriate treatment for a reasonable period of time.

> **Sample indicator D.2.1.1:** Reduction in frequency of panic attacks among patients with the diagnosis of panic disorder in a given health plan

> **Sample indicator D.2.1.2:** Stabilization of weight of patients with a new DSM-IV diagnosis of anorexia nervosa

VI. Workbook of Quality Indicators

The following workbook includes a series of indicators, measures, and standards that are presented as exemplars. Though some are based on a significant amount of research, others have not been scientifically researched. Some are more developed than others. Variation in the practicality and expense of measurement is also present. The discussion accompanying each section describes the rationale, need, and importance of the task force recommendations. Also described are the challenges, complexities, and issues raised during development of indicators, measures, and standards for the recommendation/goal. Finally, documentation from the literature is provided where appropriate.

Several methodological and practical issues should be considered in relation to all of these indicators, measures, and standards:

- These indicators, measures, and standards should be utilized with recognition of differences among cultural and ethnic groups. For example, a standard that may be appropriate in one ethnic population may not be in another.
- The definition of elements of the measures can be problematic. In many cases it is difficult to identify individuals with diagnostic or

other characteristics from a simple administrative database. In addition, certain evidence or information about types of treatment or relevant outcomes may require more extensive evaluation of medical records, or direct surveys, possibly on a sampling basis.

- In some instances, the specific designation of the standards is somewhat arbitrary. Although the overall recommendations derive from evidence-based practice guidelines, the scientific literature, and clinical consensus, there are few data available to translate these recommendations to a population-based standard. Even though strong evidence and universal agreement may exist for a particular recommendation, for example, establishing a standard must take into account that some patients may prefer not to accept particular treatment recommendations. In some cases, patients may have previous experience with treatments that have not been successful. Therefore, it is difficult to determine with accuracy how far below 100% is an acceptable standard.

- It is essential that effective methodologies for risk adjustment be developed and applied to the assessment of quality indicators. In many instances, applying the measures included in this workbook might unduly reflect negatively on programs or plans that attract and serve a high proportion of the more severely ill patients or patients with treatment-resistant conditions.

- Collection of data requires caution about matters of confidentiality. The task force's selection of indicators has been based on a principle that only aggregate data will be reported; however, some indicators may require an individual chart review to collect relevant information. The task force urges all health systems and plans to develop data collection methods that respect and protect patient confidentiality. Information that involves identification of an individual patient requires informed consent.

A. Access

A.1. Access to effective medication

Recommendation/goal A.1.1: Patients with severe and persistent mental illness should have access to newer generations of antipsychotic medications as they become available.

The new antipsychotic agents offer therapeutic advantages for many patients. Major clinical studies of schizophrenia, including the

APA practice guideline, the Expert Consensus Guidelines, the International Algorithm Project, the NIMH Patient Outcomes Research Team (PORT) for Schizophrenia recommendations, and the National Alliance for the Mentally Ill (NAMI) guidelines, indicate that new antipsychotic medications are appropriate as first-line agents in the treatment of schizophrenia. These medications are particularly recommended for patients who have an inadequate response to conventional agents or difficulty tolerating them (2).

Evidence suggests that newer-generation agents may result in improved compliance, decreased relapse rates, fewer side effects, and greater efficacy in treatment-refractory patients compared with conventional agents. (It remains possible that, with long-term use, other side effects could emerge.) The higher cost of the new antipsychotics has prompted some payers and systems of care to restrict access to them (3). Studies of the direct cost of schizophrenia show that drug therapy represents a relatively small (approximately 2%) portion of the direct medical costs. With the appearance of new, better-tolerated, but more expensive atypical antipsychotics, it is expected that the percentage spent on pharmacotherapy will rise. However, prospective, randomized studies demonstrated that patients taking atypical antipsychotics had statistically significantly better outcomes in the areas of relapse (including hospitalization), tardive dyskinesia (one-twelfth the rate), and quality of life (including return to employment and decrease in suicidal behavior) (4).

> *Sample indicator* **A.1.1:** Access to new antipsychotics for patients with schizophrenia
>
> **Sample measure A.1.1.1:** Absence of written policies that restrict first-line access or access over time
>
> **Sample standard A.1.1.1:** There should be no policy that restricts access to clinically appropriate and indicated antipsychotics.

This measure emphasizes the absence of written policies restricting first-line access. Restriction to access may not be in written policy. Pharmacy regulation takes many forms: limited or no reimbursement for medications; increased co-pay for expensive drugs; documented treatment failure on less expensive medication before a prescription for a new agent is approved; and burdensome demands on the physician (e.g., utilization review, increased documentation requirements, or more clinical assessments). In a chronic illness, access over time and first-line access are both important. Although a standard stating that there be no policy that inappropriately restricts access to new antipsychotics is warranted, it may be difficult to identify all of the ways that access is denied.

> **Sample measure A.1.1.2:** Percentage of patients in a given health plan with DSM-IV 295 diagnoses taking new antipsychotics

> **Sample standard A.1.1.2:** Current data indicate the approximate range is 20% to 40%.

The proposed numerator for the second measure is the number of adults with a diagnosis of schizophrenia (295) who received a new antipsychotic, other than clozapine (one dose or more) within the year (or other unit of time consistent with the denominator). The proposed denominator is the unduplicated number of adults (over the age of 18) with a 295 diagnosis served within the past year (or other time frame, e.g., quarter, month, during course of admission). Current data indicate that the approximate prevalence of atypical antipsychotic use ranges from 20% to 40%, but this number is increasing over time. Data are not available for establishing the definitive target percentage of patients who should be treated with these agents.

Using the unduplicated number of adults who have received any dose of an atypical agent places the emphasis on the individual patient. It identifies the proportion of patients who never receive any such trials and makes it possible to evaluate the risk factors for not receiving such a trial. In addition, it avoids overestimation of access in the case of polypharmacy. It does not, however, allow for identification of numbers of trials of these agents or for assessment of utilization of individual agents. Several other organizations—for example, the National Association of State Mental Health Program Directors (NASMHPD) and NAMI—have developed similar but not identical indicators. As an example, the NASMHPD indicator includes clozapine in its reporting. A health care plan tracking both this measure and the NASMHPD measure would have to track the number of unduplicated individuals who have received a) atypical agents other than clozapine, b) atypicals including clozapine, and c) clozapine separately.

Using the criterion of one dose or more allows for the assumption that giving one dose of an atypical agent represents a clinical decision to initiate a trial. It lends itself to measurement but does not provide information about the quality of trials once initiated (e.g., dose, duration, response, or sequence). Only standing orders for new antipsychotics should be considered (not prn orders).

In some systems, claims data may not be available. Any system without an automated pharmacy database would need to conduct a chart audit, which is time consuming and expensive. Although a sample of the patients served may improve feasibility, sampling increasingly fails to meet the expectation of accrediting bodies for complete assessment.

Recommendation/goal A.1.2: Patients with substance dependence should have access to clinically appropriate maintenance medications.

Treatment of substance dependence includes three phases: withdrawal, stabilization, and maintenance. Pharmacologic agents have been shown to be effective in the maintenance phase of treatment of opioid, alcohol, and nicotine dependence. Appropriate use of these medications decreases relapse rates and enhances recovery. On the basis of this recommendation, two sample indicators are suggested.

Opioid or Alcohol Dependence

Maintenance medications for patients with substance use disorders are used to decrease the subjective reinforcing effects of an abused substance, to make the use of an abused substance aversive, or to use an agonist substitution strategy to promote abstinence from a more dangerous illicit substance. Maintenance psychopharmacologic agents with high levels of effectiveness include methadone and LAAM (agonist medications that help some patients reduce illicit use of heroin by decreasing craving for that particular class of substances); buprenorphine (a partial opioid agonist that decreases craving for heroin); naltrexone (an opiate antagonist used as an alternative to methadone maintenance and approved for maintenance treatment of alcoholism); and disulfiram (a chemical aversion treatment that produces unpleasant but rarely lethal signs and symptoms in the presence of alcohol) (5, 6). Studies of the effectiveness of maintenance medication in the treatment of substance use disorders date back more than 30 years. In 1965, Dole and Nyswander reported that in almost all individuals who are dependent on opioids, properly prescribed methadone substantially reduced and frequently eliminated use of nonprescribed opioids (7). The database of methadone maintenance studies is larger and encompasses time periods longer than those related to any other biopsychosocial problem ever studied. Nationwide studies such as the DARP (Drug Abuse Reporting Program of Texas Christian University) study and TOPS (Treatment Outcome Prospective Study) have consistently demonstrated that illicit drug use and criminality decreased during treatment (8). New uses for maintenance medications are constantly being investigated. Further, the Substance Abuse and Mental Health Services Administration's (SAMHSA) Center for Substance Abuse Treatment recently issued best practice guidelines for the use of naltrexone in the treatment of alcoholism (9).

> *Sample indicator* **A.1.2:** Access to effective maintenance medication for patients with opioid or alcohol dependence
>
> **Sample measure A.1.2:** Percentage of adult patients in substance abuse treatment for opioid or alcohol dependence in a given health plan who are receiving one or more of the following maintenance (more than 30 days) psychopharmacological agents: methadone, buprenorphine, naltrexone, disulfiram.
>
> **Sample standard A.1.2:** Exact percentage is unknown, but a reasonable standard is estimated to be at least 20%.

The proposed numerator of the measure is the number of patients receiving maintenance medications in a given health plan. The denominator is the number of patients with a diagnosis of opioid or alcohol dependence. A reasonable standard is estimated to be 20%, but this figure is based on professional judgment and not documented in the literature. The standard probably needs to be different for alcohol or opioid dependence.

Collection of data for this indicator would require that a health plan be able to track both diagnosis and prescription information. Because methadone is given only in clinics that are federally approved, the participation of a patient might not be part of a health plan's automated prescription database. Nonetheless, there should be mention of the methadone treatment in the patient's chart. When should the data be collected? Patients may not be taking maintenance medication immediately after diagnosis or an acute treatment episode. Therefore, data should perhaps be collected 90 days after an acute episode. Tracking could be a major problem.

Nicotine Dependence

Long-term abstinence is the ultimate goal of treatment for nicotine dependence. Initial goals include moving smokers along a continuum from not contemplating smoking cessation, to contemplating smoking cessation, to initiating a quit attempt, to quitting for a short period. Psychiatrists and their patients are presented with a particular treatment challenge when the patient is admitted to a smoke-free inpatient unit and required to stop or significantly decrease the amount of smoking. Patients may have goals related to smoking that range from not contemplating cessation to wanting to use the inpatient experience as an opportunity to begin to stop smoking permanently.

Smokers with a history of anxiety, depression, or schizophrenia have particular difficulty trying to quit smoking. Several factors may contribute to this likelihood, including increased nicotine withdrawal or nicotine dependence, less social support, or fewer coping skills. Hospitalization presents a unique opportunity to manage withdrawal and provide psychosocial support for patients—regardless of their motivation to quit smoking. Since psychiatric patients appear to have more withdrawal symptomatology when they stop smoking, nicotine replacement therapy, even in early cessation attempts, is recommended (10).

Nicotine replacement therapy is used to relieve withdrawal symptoms such as anxiety, anger/irritability, depression, difficulty concentrating, and impatience. Nicotine replacement can be delivered via gum, patch, or nasal spray, depending on patient preference. Since hospitalized patients are unable to use nicotine replacement agents without a physician's order, they depend on the hospital to include it in their formulary and on their payer source to approve the expense.

> *Sample indicator* **A.1.3:** Access to effective maintenance medication for inpatients with nicotine dependence
>
> **Sample measure A.1.3:** Absence of policies that restrict access to nicotine replacement therapies, such as transdermal patches, gum, or nasal spray
>
> **Sample standard A.1.3:** 100% absence (There should be no policy that inappropriately restricts access to nicotine replacement therapies, such as transdermal patches, gum, or nasal spray.)

This measure focuses on the absence of written policies restricting access. But access may be restricted when no written policy exists; facilities may fail to include nicotine replacement in their formulary. Even if it is included in the formulary, payers may exclude it from covered expenses or create barriers to its use (e.g., complex documentation for approval). In addition, plans may simply fail to encourage primary care physicians and other clinicians to screen patients aggressively for nicotine dependence and to provide systematic interventions to aid in stopping smoking.

A.2.   Access to effective psychosocial treatment

Recommendation/goal A.2.1: Patients with severe personality disorders should have access to psychotherapy, the intensity and duration of which should be determined by the patient's clinical condition.

Borderline personality disorder (BPD) is a common and serious psychiatric disorder. Widiger and Frances (11) estimate that approximately 11% of all psychiatric outpatients and 19% of psychiatric inpatients meet diagnostic criteria for the disorder. There is increasing professional recognition that personality disorders are not as intransigent to change as once thought and that new forms of psychotherapy (e.g., dialectical behavior therapy) show promise in treating them (12). Evidence shows that patients who received intensive treatment of adequate duration demonstrate reduced severity and frequency of parasuicidal behavior and reduced need for hospitalization (13). Borderline personality disorder, if left untreated, is extraordinarily costly in terms of utilization of medical services, violence, suicide, and psychiatric hospitalization (14).

> *Sample indicator* **A.2.1:** Access to psychotherapy for patients with borderline personality disorder
>
> **Sample measure A.2.1:** Percentage of patients in a given health plan with a diagnosis of borderline personality disorder who have received psychotherapy in a given year
>
> **Sample standard A.2.1:** The exact percentage is unknown, but a reasonable standard is estimated to be at least 75% of patients with borderline personality disorder in a given health plan.

The proposed numerator for this measure is the number of patients in a given health plan with a diagnosis of 301.83 who have received psychotherapy in a given year. The denominator is the number of patients with a diagnosis of 301.83 enrolled in the same plan in the same year.

Depending on the size of the plan, the actual numbers may be small, which can lead to measurement difficulties. Underdiagnosis of BPD raises other issues.

The sample measure A.2.1 requires that a minimum number of sessions be determined that would constitute a reasonable measure of access to an appropriate course of psychotherapy. As stated in the recommendation, the intensity and duration should be determined by the patient's clinical condition. The standard of 75% of patients in a given health plan receiving psychotherapy is based on broad clinical consensus that patients with BPD should have access to psychotherapy. It accounts for the fact that some borderline patients may not agree to treatment and others may not need psychotherapy in any given year.

A.3. Access to appropriate specialized services

Recommendation/goal A.3.1: ECT should be an available treatment option.

Electroconvulsive therapy (ECT) has a high rate of therapeutic success, relative speed in ameliorating depressive symptoms, and an excellent safety profile. It should be considered as an initial treatment for severe major depression accompanied by psychotic features, catatonic stupor, severe suicidality, and food refusal leading to nutritional compromise, as well as in other situations where rapid antidepressant response is required. ECT is also indicated as a first-line treatment for patients who have previously shown a preferential response to this treatment modality or who prefer it. It should be considered for all depressed patients with functional impairment whose illness has not responded to medication or who have a medical condition that precludes the use of antidepressant medications (15). ECT has been in continuous use for almost 60 years, and its safety and efficacy have been documented by the National Institutes of Health, the APA, the U.S. Agency for Health Care Policy and Research (AHCPR), the British Royal College of Psychiatrists, and similar professional organizations around the world (16). Hermann and colleagues (17) determined that the rates of ECT use are highly variable, greater than for most medical and surgical procedures.

Sample indicator **A.3.1:** Availability of ECT to patients for whom it is clinically indicated

Sample measure A.3.1: Documentation of a capacity within an organized system of care, through a network or by contract arrangement, to provide ECT to patients for whom it is clinically indicated

Sample standard A.3.1: 100% of organized systems of care should have demonstrable capacity to provide ECT to patients for whom it is clinically indicated.

The sample measure seeks to verify the capacity of a given system of care to provide ECT to patients who need it. However, this measure cannot ensure that patients who can actually benefit from ECT have the option of receiving it, because there may be other administrative and procedural barriers to accessing it.

Recommendation/goal A.3.2: Children and adolescents should have access to appropriate psychiatric evaluation and treatment services.

Evaluation of children and adolescents requires knowledge of normal and pathological development, as well as familiarity with the range of general medical and psychiatric conditions that affect individuals at different ages. Psychiatric evaluation of children and adolescents requires experience in specific interview and other assessment techniques (18, 19).

Sample indicator **A.3.2:** Availability of appropriate specialized services for prepubertal children with depression in a given health plan

Sample measure A.3.2: Percentage of prepubertal children with depressive disorder or dysthymia in a given health plan who receive specialized services from a provider with appropriate training and expertise

Sample standard A.3.2: An estimated 90% of all prepubertal children with a diagnosis of major depressive disorder or dysthymia in a given health plan

The proposed numerator for this measure is the number of children, age 12 and under, in a given health plan with a diagnosis of major depression or dysthymia who have seen a health professional with specialized training and/or expertise. The proposed denominator is the number of prepubertal children with one of these diagnoses in a given health plan.

Health plans would need a mechanism to identify health professionals who have appropriate specialized training and/or expertise across a full range of health professionals. The plan's data retrieval system should be capable of identifying the numerator and denominator. The measure does not address the frequent problem of under-recognition of children with psychiatric disorders, but it is one method of learning whether access to specialized services is available.

B.   Quality

B.1.   Comprehensive evaluation

Recommendation/goal B.1.1: Patients with new onset of cognitive impairment need a comprehensive assessment that rules out treatable causes of that impairment.

Patients with a new onset of cognitive impairment require a thorough diagnostic evaluation. The evaluation serves to identify a diagnosis that may guide specific treatment decisions and to reveal any treatable psychiatric or general medical conditions (e.g., major depression, thyroid disease, B_{12} deficiency, tertiary syphilis, hydrocephalus, or structural brain lesion) that might be causing or exacerbating the dementia. Detailed descriptions of the elements of such a diagnostic evaluation have been identified in documents such as the Consensus Conference on the Differential Diagnosis of Dementing Disorders of the National Institute on Aging, National Institute of Neurological Disorders and Stroke, National Institute of Mental Health, and the National Institutes of Health (20); the practice guideline on the diagnosis and evaluation of dementia of the American Academy of Neurology (21); and the AHCPR's Clinical Practice Guideline on Recognition and Initial Assessment of Alzheimer's Disease and Related Dementias (22). General principles of psychiatric evaluation are outlined in the APA's *Practice Guideline for Psychiatric Evaluation of Adults* (23). The APA practice guideline recommends the following evaluative tests: a review of the patient's medications; laboratory studies (i.e., complete blood count, blood chemistry battery [including glucose, electrolytes, calcium, and kidney and liver function tests]), measurement of vitamin B_{12} level, syphilis serology, thyroid function tests, and determination of erythrocyte sedimentation rate. Failure to assess and diagnose the cognitively impaired patient accurately could be catastrophic because it could condemn the patient to irreversible dementia.

Sample indicator **B.1.1:** Assessment of cognitive impairment for individuals with new onset of symptoms

Sample measure B.1.1: Percentage of patients in a given health plan with new-onset cognitive impairment who receive a medical workup that includes a sequence of evaluative tests until a positive finding (if found) indicates a potential cause of new-onset cognitive impairment

Sample standard B.1.1: Goal should be 100% of people about whom questions of cognitive impairment have been raised

The numerator proposed for this measure is the number of patients who present with new-onset cognitive impairment who, within 30 days of evaluation, have received the specific diagnostic tests documented in the APA practice guideline. The denominator is the number of patients newly diagnosed with dementia (290.00–290.99). A sample of patients with new-onset dementia generally cannot be determined precisely using administrative databases but could be estimated using the following definition: patients continuously enrolled for 2 years who did not have a claim reflecting a diagnosis of dementia in year one but did have such a claim in year two. The denominator could be inaccurate if the diagnosis is missed or erroneous. Data collection would require medical record review and significant subjective judgment to determine whether a sequence of tests and evaluation of positive results were done. Because of poor organization, illegibility, and omissions, medical records may not be an adequate data source. Alternatively, a separate data collection system (e.g., a brief questionnaire) could be employed. A standard of 100% is suggested because the consequences of a missed diagnosis are potentially devastating (24).

B.2. Appropriate use of medications

Recommendation/goal B.2.1: Medications should be used in appropriate dosage and duration for those disorders for which they have been shown to be effective.

A wide variety of medications have been well documented for the treatment of specific mental disorders. Because of the breadth of this recommendation, two possible indicators are highlighted.

Major Depressive Disorder

During the past 30 years, significant progress in basic and clinical research has led to the development of new generations of antidepressants with increased efficacy and decreased side effects. These developments have led to better tolerance and acceptance by patients. The selection and adjustment of the antidepressant agent and dose take into consideration the medication's side-effect profile and typically effective dose range, as well as the patient's age and health status. Continuation treatment is administered to prevent relapse during the period following symptomatic recovery. The available data indicate that patients treated for a first episode of uncomplicated depression who exhibit a satisfactory response to an antidepressant agent should continue a full therapeutic dose of that agent for at least 16–20 weeks after achieving full remission. Patients who have a history of recurrent or severe depression may need maintenance treatment of more than 20 weeks (15).

> *Sample indicator* **B.2.1:** Current treatment with an antidepressant medication of patients with major depressive disorder, moderate or severe
>
> **Sample measure B.2.1:** Percentage of patients in a given health plan with major depressive disorder, moderate or severe, receiving an appropriate dose of antidepressant medication
>
> **Sample standard B.2.1:** Estimate 75% of patients with major depressive disorder, moderate or severe

The proposed numerator is the number of patients diagnosed as above, receiving an appropriate dose of antidepressant medication. The proposed denominator of the measure is the number of patients in a given health plan with a diagnosis of major depressive disorder, moderate or severe. Although dose ranges are suggested for all antidepressants, the term *appropriate* needs definition. Some plans have pharmacy databases that are able to correlate dose, drug, and diagnosis, but for those that do not, data collection would require chart review. The indicators, as currently written, do not account for the appropriate duration of treatment detailed in the recommendation. For patients who receive maintenance treatment, the optimal duration of such treatment will vary with patient characteristics. The suggested standard of 75% is based on clinical judgment and may need to be refined.

Bipolar Disorder

Bipolar I disorder affects approximately 0.8% of the adult population. Pharmacologic agents are a critical component in the treatment of patients with bipolar disorder. The primary treatment of either a manic or a depressive episode in a patient with bipolar disorder involves the use of a mood-stabilizing medication. Three mood stabilizers—lithium, valproic acid, and carbamazepine—have been shown to be effective in the treatment of acute episodes (25).

> *Sample indicator* **B.2.2:** Current treatment with a mood stabilizer of patients with bipolar I disorder
>
> **Sample measure B.2.2:** Percentage of patients in a given health plan with bipolar I disorder, in an acute episode, receiving valproic acid, lithium, or carbamazepine
>
> **Sample standard B.2.2:** Estimate 90% of patients in manic or depressed episode

The proposed numerator of the measure is the number of patients in a given health plan who are receiving valproic acid, lithium, or carbamazepine. The proposed denominator is the total number of patients in a given health plan diagnosed with bipolar I disorder in acute episode. Coding systems may not be sensitive enough to distinguish patients experiencing an acute episode, which occurs in the course of a long-term illness. Data retrieval would require a database that tracks diagnosis as well as prescription data. Such a system would indicate which patients were prescribed a mood stabilizer but would not verify which were actually receiving it. Chart review may more accurately identify patients who reported taking the medication but would be resource intensive. It is likely that the number of patients meeting review criteria in any given database would be relatively small. The estimate of 90%, as identified in the standard, may need to be refined. Not all patients, because of preference, stability, or intolerance to medications, would necessarily need to be receiving new medications, but the precise size of that group cannot be determined. In addition, some patients may be well treated with mood stabilizers other than those mentioned here.

B.3. Appropriate use of psychosocial treatments

Recommendation/goal B.3.1: Psychotherapy, psychiatric rehabilitation, and other psychosocial treatments should be used in appropriate intensity and duration in treating disorders for which they have been shown to be effective.

Programs of Assertive Community Treatment (PACT) have demonstrated effectiveness for persons with severe and persistent mental illness, here defined as individuals with major mental illness on Axis I who are unstable. Reviews of first- and second-generation controlled studies of the PACT model consistently found the model to be more effective than traditional interventions in reducing days spent in psychiatric inpatient settings. PACT demonstrated advantages in bolstering clinical stability, independent living, and satisfaction outcomes among clients (26). Relative to usual community care, PACT for homeless persons with severe and persistent mental illness shift the locus of care from crisis-oriented services to ongoing outpatient care and produce better housing, clinical, and life-satisfaction outcomes (27). Studies of cost-effectiveness have demonstrated savings when compared with traditional service provision (28, 29, 30).

Criteria for programs that meet the operational definition of PACT include the following: a) service in the community, not just the clinic office; b) assertive engagement/outreach; c) small caseload (client-clinician ratio of approximately 10:1); d) team approach; e) multidisciplinary team, including at least one psychiatrist, nurse, and substance abuse specialist; f) continuous responsibility; g) continuity of staffing; h) intensity of contact (high level of service when needed); and i) close work with support team (family, employers, landlords, etc.) (31).

Sample indicator **B.3.1:** Appropriate use of psychosocial treatment for severely and persistently mentally ill patients

Sample measure B.3.1: Proportion of severely and persistently mentally ill patients with greater than or equal to two inpatient stays and/or four ER/crisis visits in past 12 months, in a given health plan, who are enrolled in PACT

Sample standard B.3.1: Greater than 50%

The numerator proposed for this measure is the number of adults with a diagnosis of schizophrenia (295) who have had two or more inpatient stays and/or four ER/crisis visits in the past 12 months who are enrolled in PACT. The denominator is the number of adult patients with a 295 diagnosis and two or more inpatient stays and/or four ER crisis visits in the past 12 months. Although this standard is proposed as an appropriate indicator, there are no data that directly inform the question of the number of treatment engagements that would identify an individual as a high user of services and therefore qualified as a candidate for PACT.

The operational definition of PACT needs to be clear, since some programs offer some but not all the services of traditional PACT and some programs offer all the services of PACT but do not call themselves a PACT. Careful assessment of whether PACT meet established criteria would increase the validity of the measure but would complicate assessment. In many plans, ER/crisis visits are not reimbursed (or documented in databases) unless they result in hospitalization. This leads to underestimation of the size of the population of individuals who are unstable and in need of increased services such as PACT. Potential data sources include administrative claims data, contract reporting systems, Medicaid management information systems, and various provider information systems. Even if the data were recorded, retrieval and tracking would be very complex and labor intensive. The measure suggested for the sample standard (greater than 50%) is reasonable but arbitrary.

B.4. Appropriate use of screening/prevention services

Recommendation/goal B.4.1: Inquiries should be made about the status and functioning of children of parents with psychiatric disorders associated with significant dysfunction.

Several risk factors have been associated with the etiology and pathogenesis of psychiatric disorders in children of psychiatrically ill parents. Both genetic and environmental factors may contribute to an increased risk of psychiatric disorders and impairment in these children. Early screening could be a means of identifying the early signs and symptoms of psychopathology or impairment in the child's functioning at home or school so that early treatment could be provided. Interventions to improve parenting skills, foster greater family stability, and provide psychoeducation to the child and parents may help to prevent or decrease the impact of the parent's illness on children and families identified as at risk (32, 33).

Sample indicator **B.4.1:** Screening of children at risk for psychiatric disorders in a given health plan

Sample measure B.4.1: Use of standardized instruments, clinical examination, or other methods (e.g., Child Behavior Checklist) to screen children at risk for psychiatric disorders (e.g., children of parents with diagnosed psychiatric disorders)

Sample standard B.4.1: Goal should be the majority of children at risk.

The proposed numerator of the measure is the number of children at risk who are screened. The proposed denominator is the total number of children at risk. The phrase used in the sample indicator "children at risk for psychiatric disorders" needs to be defined to identify the numerator and the denominator. Measurement issues arise over the method of identification; informed consent and confidentiality; responsibility for identification and screening; placement of recorded data to permit retrieval; and interpretation and use of screening results. There are no data to suggest what an acceptable sample standard should be.

Recommendation/goal B.4.2: Patients receiving psychiatric evaluations should be explicitly asked about current substance use and evaluated for the presence and/or history of substance use disorders.

Psychiatric evaluation involves a systematic consideration of several broad domains, including history of substance use. The psychoactive substance use history includes past and present use of both licit and illicit psychoactive substances—the quantity and frequency of use and route of administration; the pattern of use; functional interpersonal or legal consequences of use; tolerance and withdrawal phenomena; and any temporal association between substance use and present psychiatric illness (23). Inclusion of this domain of evaluation is based on the frequency with which substance use disorders are associated with other forms of psychopathology. Treatment-seeking patients tend to be at the higher end of the range. Approximately one-third of hospitalized psychiatric patients manifest comorbid non-nicotine substance use disorders (5).

Sample indicator **B.4.2:** Screening of patients for substance use disorders

Sample measure B.4.2: Percentage of patients in a given health plan receiving psychiatric evaluations whose records indicate explicit evidence of assessment, by history or formal measure, of current and/or past substance use disorders

Sample standard B.4.2: Estimate 90% of patients 15 years or older

The proposed numerator of the measure is the number of patients receiving psychiatric evaluations who are assessed for substance use disorders. The denominator is the total number of patients who receive psychiatric evaluations. Depending on the system of care, this information may not be routinely available in standard administrative data sets. Data collection would require chart review as well as a way of identifying all patients who had received a psychiatric evaluation. The term used in the sample measure *explicit evidence of assessment* needs to be defined. The sample standard of 90% of patients 15 years or older is based on clinical judgment.

C.   Perceptions of Care

C.1.   Patient

Recommendation/goal C.1.1: Health care systems or plans should regularly and systematically solicit information from their patients about their perceptions and experiences of the care provided.

It is an intrinsically desirable end for patients to have positive experiences of their care. It is important to learn as much as possible about the patient's perception of care, both positive and negative. It is also valuable for recruitment and retention of plan subscribers and for risk management. Patients can be an important source of information regarding interpersonal aspects of health care quality. Dissatisfaction with care has been associated with poor patient adherence to treatment, changing clinicians, disenrollment from health plans, and worse patient-reported outcomes (34). The patient's perception of care has been widely adopted as an integral component of health care quality assessment and clinical quality improvement.

> *Sample indicator* **C.1.1:** Assessment of patients' perceptions of care
>
> **Sample measure C.1.1:** Use of standardized questionnaires to gather data on a representative population sample on patients' perceptions of care
>
> **Sample standard C.1.1:** 100% of plans will use standardized questionnaires to gather data on patients' perceptions of care

Use of standardized surveys is increasingly required by federal and state agencies for public sector patients and by accreditation organizations for patients treated in the private sector (35). A representative sample of all patients should be surveyed at least annually, with completion rates of at least 40%. Data should be analyzed and distributed to management and clinical staff and made publicly available.

Patient surveys provide better information about interpersonal quality than technical quality of care. Patient characteristics (e.g., age, gender, physical and mental health status) can bias patient perceptions of health care quality, resulting in lower ratings that are unrelated to the quality of care received (36, 37). Higher survey response rates minimize bias.

Measures need to be psychometrically validated and reliable and employed with a representative sample of patients. Because use of the measure (not degree of satisfaction) is the standard, comparability of instruments is less critical. Limitations to assessing patient satisfaction are related to the institution's resources available to collect, analyze, and act on satisfaction data, and to willingness and ability of the patient/beneficiary population to respond to the survey. Experiences with response rates of patient surveys in a variety of clinical settings and health plans suggest that a 40% response rate is an achievable goal. The difficulty that plans or service settings encounter in meeting the standard of 40% will depend on the sociodemographic and clinical status of their patient populations.

C.2. Family

Recommendation/goal C.2.1: When families are involved in treatment, health care systems or plans should regularly and systematically solicit information from families about their perceptions and experiences of the care provided.

Family perception of the care received by their family member may or may not be the same as the patient's perception of care. Families are an important source of information regarding interpersonal aspects of health care quality. Their perspective is an integral component of health care quality assessment and clinical quality improvement. The perspective of families is of critical importance in the treatment of children and adolescents, the severely and persistently mentally ill, the developmentally disordered, the elderly, and patients with dementia. Although family perception should not replace data from the patient's perspective, it should be used to enrich the overall view of clinical care (38).

Sample indicator **C.2.1:** Assessment of families' perceptions of care

Sample measure C.2.1: When families are involved in treatment, standardized questionnaires should be used to assess families' perceptions of care.

Sample standard C.2.1: 100% of plans will use standardized questionnaires to assess families' perceptions of care.

The measure proposes that when families are involved in treatment, health care plans will use standardized questionnaires 100% of the time to assess families' perceptions of care. The term *involved in treatment* requires definition since such involvement may vary tremendously. Access to families may be difficult, and identifying the family member who is able to give the most informed feedback may prove problematic. Confidentiality issues are complicated. Little research data are available to suggest how family information can be used most effectively to influence quality of care. The instruments used in assessing family perceptions are not well developed. There is little information to demonstrate what response rate is achievable. If response rates are low, bias is a significant concern.

C.3. Clinician

Recommendation/goal C.3.1: Health care systems or plans should regularly and systematically solicit information from individual clinicians providing care within their organizations about their perceptions and experiences of the care provided by the organization.

> *Sample indicator* **C.3.1:** Assessment of clinicians' perceptions of care
>
> **Sample measure C.3.1:** Use by a health care system or a plan of systematic independent methods to survey individual system providers' perceptions of their capacity to provide appropriate care within the system
>
> **Sample standard C.3.1:** 100% of plans must use independent methods to survey providers' perceptions of their capacity to provide appropriate treatment within the system.

This indicator has not been reported in the literature. However, it is considered essential that the clinician's perception of his or her capacity to provide appropriate care within the system be systematically assessed. For this reason, the indicator is included and the field is challenged to develop measurement methods.

D. Outcome

D.1. Improved level of functioning and quality of life, and minimization of social and economic cost

Recommendation/goal D.1.1: Many patients with mental illness that significantly impairs functioning should be able to resume some degree of productive occupational or educational activity after receiving treatment known to be effective for their conditions.

An important quality outcome indicator is functional status. Most persons with severe and persistent mental illness have impaired functioning in multiple life areas, including employment, interpersonal relationships, self-care, and community living skills (use of transportation, money management, etc.). Perhaps one of the most uniform consequences of severe mental illness is a vastly compromised capacity for productive activity. A distinctive characteristic of schizophrenia is unemployment. Virtually all clients with severe mental illness who are in rehabilitation programs have significant vocational impairments, and most are not employed at any given point in time (39). However, the clear majority of persons with severe mental illnesses identify paid employment as one of their goals (40).

Although available medical treatments effectively reduce clinical symptoms for many individuals, functional impairments often remain. These residual disabilities constitute substantial impediments for patients and are typically identified by patients and families as major priorities for improving their quality of life. The severe personal and family disruption in functioning associated with schizophrenia is mirrored in the social and economic cost associated with the illness (41). There is growing evidence that certain types of rehabilitation influence not only the patient's ability to participate in paid or volunteer work, to care for a home, or to participate in a training or school program, but also treatment adherence and symptom reduction, functional status in other areas (activities of daily living, maintenance of living situation, etc.), self-esteem, and subjective quality of life (42).

Sample indicator **D.1.1:** Resumption of productive activities by patients with severe and persistent mental illness when no longer in the acute phase of illness

Sample measure D.1.1: Percentage of patients in a given health plan with a DSM-IV diagnosis of schizophrenia or schizoaffective disorder in stabilization phase of illness involved (greater than or equal to 2 days per week) in one or more of the following:

1. Paid or volunteer work
2. Child care or homemaking
3. Rehabilitation or day program and/or school

Sample standard D.1.1: Estimate 80% of patients will show some resumption of productive activities in one or more of the areas noted above.

The proposed numerator of the measure is the number of patients in a given health plan with a DSM-IV diagnosis of schizophrenia or schizoaffective disorder (one example of severe and persistent mental illness) in a stabilization phase of the disorder who are involved at least 2 days a week in one or more specified activities (paid or volunteer work, child care or homemaking, rehabilitation or day program, and/or school). The denominator is all patients in a given health plan with the same DSM-IV diagnosis who are in a stabilization phase of the disorder. The information may be difficult and expensive to collect because it may not be clearly documented and would require chart review. The proposed standard of 80% is an estimate because there are no clear target standards for what a high-quality system can achieve. The standard also mixes participation in rehabilitative services with work and homemaking, since the majority of patients can benefit from rehabilitation services and current data suggest many patients (probably well over 50%) do not receive these services.

D.2. Reduction and/or stabilization of symptoms/signs

Recommendation/goal D.2.1: Patients receiving treatment known to be effective for their conditions should experience a significant reduction in symptoms and signs after receiving appropriate treatment for a reasonable period of time.

The outcome of treatment for psychiatric conditions can be measured in quantifiable terms. The sample indicators below focus on panic disorder and anorexia nervosa. The unit of measurement in panic disorder is the number of panic attacks within a defined period of time compared with the number of attacks before treatment. The measurement in anorexia nervosa is the patient's weight before and after psychiatric intervention.

Panic Disorder

Panic disorder is a common psychiatric illness that can have a chronic course and be associated with significant morbidity. The care of patients with panic disorder involves a comprehensive array of approaches that are designed to reduce the frequency and severity of panic episodes, reduce morbidity, and improve patient functioning. Modalities for which there is considerable evidence of efficacy in the treatment of panic disorder include psychotherapy, specifically cognitive-behavioral therapy (CBT), and pharmacotherapy. At the end of successful treatment, the patient should have markedly fewer and less intense panic attacks than before treatment (41). Comorbid psychiatric illness, concurrent general medical illnesses, and certain demographic or psychosocial features of patients with panic disorder may have important influences on treatment and must be considered in treatment planning and evaluation of outcomes (43).

> *Sample indicator* **D.2.1.1:** Reduction in frequency of panic attacks among patients with the diagnosis of panic disorder in a given health plan

> **Sample measure D.2.1.1:** Number of panic attacks in a given time interval compared with a pretreatment interval

> **Sample standard D.2.1.1:** Estimate 75% of patients will show a reduction in the number of panic attacks within 6 months.

The numerator suggested for the measure is the number of panic attacks reported by the patient during a 2-week interval 6 months after the initiation of treatment. The denominator is the number of panic attacks reported by the patient during a 2-week interval before treatment began. Patients may not be able to document the pretreatment number accurately, and this may not routinely be documented in the medical record. Data retrieval would require review of the medical record or maintenance of a separate data system. Consideration must be given to the most appropriate time to measure improvement. The current measure suggests data collection at 6 months in order to document sustained improvement. A limitation to using the 6-month point is that patients often realize full treatment benefit in shorter periods of time and may not still be in treatment at 6 months. The standard, 75% of patients showing a reduction in the number of panic attacks within 6 months, is an estimate based on reported efficacy of various types of treatment. It requires further refinement.

Anorexia Nervosa

Anorexia nervosa is characterized by inability to maintain a minimal normal body weight (85%) for age and height, intense fear of gaining weight or becoming fat even though underweight, distorted body image, and amenorrhea (DSM-IV, p. 539). The prevalence of eating disorders appears to be increasing and may range from 1% to 4% of adolescent and young adult women in predominantly white upper-middle-class and middle-class student groups. Increasing numbers of cases are being seen in males, minorities, and women of all age groups. Follow-up studies conducted at least 4 years after onset of illness show that about 44% of patients had an overall good outcome (weight restored to within 15% of recommended weight and regular menstruation established), about 24% had poor outcome (weight was never adequately restored), 28% had an intermediate outcome, and 5% had died (44).

Treatment interventions are first aimed at nutritional rehabilitation and the restoration of normal eating patterns to correct the biological and psychological sequelae of malnutrition. Consensus currently exists that many of the physical and psychological symptoms of eating disorders may result from malnutrition. A reasonable rate of weight gain is thought to be between 1 to 3 pounds per week in an inpatient setting and ½ to 2 pounds per week in an outpatient setting. The concurrent longer-term goals are to diagnose and help resolve the psychological, family, social, and behavioral problems that frequently accompany the disorder so that relapse does not occur (44).

> *Sample indicator* **D.2.1.2:** Stabilization of weight of patients with a new DSM-IV diagnosis of anorexia nervosa

> **Sample measure D.2.1.2:** Percentage of patients who are able to achieve and sustain a normal weight within 6 months after receiving a DSM-IV diagnosis of anorexia nervosa

> **Sample standard D.2.1.2:** Exact standard not known; will depend in part on definition of normal weight and severity of patient population; estimate at least 50%

The numerator suggested for the measure is the number of patients with a new diagnosis of anorexia nervosa who are able to achieve and sustain a normal weight within 6 months after receiving the diagnosis. The denominator is the number of patients within the identified population with a new diagnosis of anorexia nervosa. The determination of a normal weight is highly individualized and needs to be clearly identified in the medical record. Patients may drop out of treatment or change providers over a 6-month period. The number of patients with a new anorexia nervosa diagnosis may be very small. Data collection would require that a system be able to identify and track this diagnosis over time, along with individual chart review. The sample standard of 50% is an estimate.

VII. Next Steps

The recently created APA Office of Quality Improvement and Psychiatric Services enhances the APA's efforts, first, to document the scientific basis of psychiatric care through the development of practice guidelines, and second, to advocate for strong standards for quality care through accreditation and related processes. The overall mission of the office is to facilitate the optimal provision of quality psychiatric services, including substance abuse services. Two important goals are

- To promote the use of scientifically valid data and accumulated clinical experience to inform the processes of clinical and policy decision making; and
- To provide psychiatric leadership in the improvement of treatment by developing, commenting on, and disseminating quality improvement measures for use by clinicians, organized systems of care, accrediting bodies, and others.

The Council on Quality Improvement provides a venue for this work within the APA. The council includes the Steering Committee on Practice Guidelines; Committee on Standards and Survey Procedures; Committee on Quality Indicators (the sequel to this task force); and Task Force on Quality Indicators for Children.

A critical component of all of the efforts related to quality improvement is the ongoing development of indicators, or measures, that accurately and appropriately reflect important aspects of the quality of care. In addition to the ongoing work of the Council on Quality Improvement, three particular efforts are as follows.

Promotion and Implementation of Quality of Care Indicators

The new Committee on Quality Indicators will review comments on this report and suggestions for additional indicators. In conjunction with the council and its other components, the committee will also develop strategies to disseminate the indicators, encourage additional research, and promote adoption of the quality indicators by oversight organizations that are implementing measurement programs.

Disorder-Specific Quality of Care Indicators

Under the direction of the Steering Committee on Practice Guidelines, key recommendations and related measures are being developed for each practice guideline. These recommendations are evidence based and provide a method for assessing the quality of care for patients with specific disorders.

Task Force on Child and Adolescent Quality Indicators

A task force has been established that will develop a framework and set of indicators that address specific quality issues for the population of children and adolescents with mental disorders. These efforts will extend the work of the Task Force on Quality Indicators by addressing issues that are particularly important for this special and often underserved population.

References

1. Eddy DM: Performance measurement: problems and solutions. Health Aff (Millwood) 17(4):7–25, 1998
2. American Psychiatric Association: Practice guideline for the treatment of patients with schizophrenia. Am J Psychiatry 154 (4, suppl):1–63, 1997
3. Lehman AF, Steinwachs DM: At Issue: Translating research into practice: the Schizophrenia Patient Outcomes Research Team (PORT) treatment recommendations. Schizophr Bull 24(1):1–10, 1998
4. Haveman, JK: Access to atypical antipsychotics: a public payor's perspective. Behavioral Healthcare Tomorrow 7(4):45–48, 1998
5. American Psychiatric Association: Practice guideline for the treatment of patients with substance use disorders: alcohol, cocaine, opioids. Am J Psychiatry 152 (11, suppl):1–59, 1995
6. National Consensus Development Panel on Effective Medical Treatment of Opiate Addiction: Effective medical treatment of opiate addiction. JAMA 280(22):1936–1943, 1998
7. Dole VP, Nyswander ME: A medical treatment for diacetylmorphine (heroin) addiction: a clinical trial with methadone hydrochloride. JAMA 193:646–650, 1965
8. Senay E: Opioids: methadone maintenance, in The American Psychiatric Press Textbook of Substance Abuse Treatment. Edited by Galanter M, Kleber HD. Washington, DC, American Psychiatric Press, 1994, pp 209–222
9. Substance Abuse and Mental Health Services Administration, Center for Substance Abuse Treatment: Naltrexone and Alcoholism Treatment (Treatment Improvement Protocol Series 28). Rockville, MD, Substance Abuse and Mental Health Services Administration, October 26, 1998
10. American Psychiatric Association: Practice guideline for the treatment of patients with nicotine dependence. Am J Psychiatry 153 (10, suppl):1–31, 1996
11. Widiger TA, Frances AJ: Epidemiology, diagnosis, and comorbidity of borderline personality disorder, in American Psychiatric Press Review of Psychiatry, Vol 8. Edited by Tasman A, Hales RE, Frances AJ. Washington, DC, American Psychiatric Press, 1989, pp 8–25
12. Gabbard G: Psychotherapy of personality disorders. Journal of Practical Psychiatry and Behavioral Health 3:327–333, 1997

13. Linehan MM, Armstrong HE, Suarez A, Allmon D, Heard HL: Cognitive-behavioral treatment of chronically parasuicidal borderline patients. Arch Gen Psychiatry 48(12):1060–1064, 1991

14. Sabo AN, Gunderson JG, Najavits LM, Chauncey D, Kisiel C: Changes in self-destructiveness of borderline patients in psychotherapy. J Nerv Ment Dis 183(6):370–376, 1995

15. American Psychiatric Association: Practice guideline for major depressive disorder in adults. Am J Psychiatry 150 (4, suppl):1–26, 1993

16. American Psychiatric Association Task Force on Electroconvulsive Therapy: The Practice of Electroconvulsive Therapy. Washington, DC, American Psychiatric Association, 1990

17. Hermann RC, Dorwart RA, Hoover CW, Brody J: Variation in ECT use in the United States. Am J Psychiatry 152(6):869–875, 1995

18. King RA: Practice parameters for the psychiatric assessment of children and adolescents. J Am Acad Child Adolesc Psychiatry 36 (10, suppl):4S-20S, 1997

19. Practice parameters for the assessment and treatment of children and adolescents with depressive disorders. AACAP. J Am Acad Child Adolesc Psychiatry 37 (10, suppl):63S–83S, 1998

20. NIH Consensus Development Panel on the Differential Diagnosis of Dementing Diseases: Differential diagnosis of dementing diseases. JAMA 258:3411–3416, 1987

21. Okagaki JF, Alter M, Byrne TN, Daube JR, Franklin G, Frishberg BM, Goldstein ML, Greenberg MK, Lanska DJ, Mishra S, Odenheimer GL, Paulson G, Pearl RA, Rosenberg JH, Sila C, Stevens JC: Practice parameter for the diagnosis and evaluation of dementia. Neurology 44:2203–2206, 1994

22. Agency for Health Care Policy and Research: Recognition and Initial Assessment of Alzheimer's Disease and Related Dementias (Clinical Guideline No 19; AHCPR Publ No 97-0702). Washington, DC, U.S. Department of Health and Human Services, November 1996

23. American Psychiatric Association: Practice guideline for psychiatric evaluation of adults. Am J Psychiatry 152 (11, suppl):63–80, 1995

24. American Psychiatric Association: Practice guideline for the treatment of patients with Alzheimer's disease and other dementias of late life. Am J Psychiatry 154 (5, suppl):1–39, 1997

25. American Psychiatric Association: Practice guideline for the treatment of patients with bipolar disorder. Am J Psychiatry 151 (12, suppl):1–36, 1994

26. Burns BJ, Santos AB: Assertive community treatment: an update of randomized trials. Psychiatr Serv 46(7):669–675, 1995

27. Lehman AF, Dixon LB, Kernan E, DeForge BR, Postrado LT: A randomized trial of assertive community treatment for homeless persons with severe mental illness. Arch Gen Psychiatry 54(11):1038–1043, 1997

28. Essock SM, Frisman LK, Kontos NJ: Cost-effectiveness of assertive community treatment teams. Am J Orthopsychiatry 68(2):179–190, 1998

29. Knapp M, Beecham J, Koutsogeorgopoulou V, Hallam A, Fenyo A, Marks IM, Connolly J, Audini B, Muijen M: Service use and costs of home-based versus hospital-based care for people with serious mental illness. Br J Psychiatry 165(2):195–203, 1994

30. Rosenheck R, Neale M, Leaf P, Milstein R, Frisman L: Multisite experimental cost study of intensive psychiatric community care. Schizophr Bull 21(1):129–140, 1995

31. Teague GB, Drake RE, Ackerson TH: Evaluating use of continuous treatment teams for persons with mental illness and substance abuse. Psychiatr Serv 46(7):689–695, 1995

32. Beardslee WR, Salt P, Porterfield K, Rothberg PC, van de Velde P, Swatling S, Hoke L, Moilanen DL: Comparison of preventive interventions for families with parental affective disorder. J Am Acad Child Adolesc Psychiatry 32(2):254–263, 1993

33. Silverman MM: Children of psychiatrically ill parents: a prevention perspective. Hosp Community Psychiatry 40(12):1257–1265, 1989

34. Kaplan S, Ware J: The patient's role in health care and quality assessment, in Producing Quality Care: Future Challenges. Edited by Gnan DB. Ann Arbor, MI, Health Administration Press, 1995, pp 25–69

35. Cleary PD, Edgman-Levitan S: Health care quality: incorporating consumer perspectives. JAMA 278(19):1608–1612, 1997

36. Hermann RC, Ettner SL, Dorwart RA: The influence of psychiatric disorders on patients' ratings of satisfaction with health care. Med Care 36(5): 720–727, 1998

37. Cleary PD, McNeil BJ: Patient satisfaction as an indicator of quality care. Inquiry 25:25–36, 1988

38. Sederer LI, Dickey B: Outcomes Assessment in Clinical Practice. Baltimore, MD, Williams & Wilkins, 1996

39. Attkisson C, Cook J, Karno M, Lehman A, McGlashan TH, Meltzer HY, O'Connor M, Richardson D, Rosenblatt A, Wells K, et al: Clinical services research. Schizophr Bull 18(4):561–626, 1992

40. Rogers ES, Walsh D, Massotta L, Danley K: Massachusetts Survey of Client Preferences for Community Support Programs: Final Report. Unpublished manuscript, Center for Psychosocial Rehabilitation, Boston, MA, 1991

41. Rupp A, Keith SJ: The costs of schizophrenia: assessing the burden. Psychiatr Clin North Am 16(2):413–423, 1993

42. Lehman AF: Vocational rehabilitation in schizophrenia. Schizophr Bull 21(4):645–656, 1995

43. American Psychiatric Association: Practice guideline for the treatment of patients with panic disorder. Am J Psychiatry 155 (5, suppl):1–34, 1998

44. American Psychiatric Association: Practice guideline for eating disorders. Am J Psychiatry 151 (12, suppl):1–36, 1994

Acronyms and Abbreviations

AACAP	American Academy of Child and Adolescent Psychiatry
AAHCC	American Accreditation Healthcare Commission
AHCPR	Agency for Health Care Policy and Research
AMAP	American Medical Accreditation Program
APA	American Psychiatric Association
BHMAP	Behavioral Health Measurement Advisory Panel
BPD	Borderline personality disorder
CBT	Cognitive-behavioral therapies
CQI	Continuous quality improvement
DARP	Drug Abuse Reporting Program
ECT	Electroconvulsive therapy
HEDIS	Healthplan Employer Data and Information Set
JCAHO	Joint Commission on Accreditation of Healthcare Organizations
NAMI	National Alliance for the Mentally Ill
NASMHPD	National Association of State Mental Health Program Directors
NCQA	National Committee for Quality Assurance
NIH	National Institutes of Health
NIMH	National Institute of Mental Health
ORYX	Not an acronym but refers to JCAHO's performance measurement program
PACT	Programs of Assertive Community Treatment
PMCC	Performance Measurement Coordinating Council
PORT	Patient Outcomes Research Team
SAMHSA	Substance Abuse and Mental Health Services Administration
TIP	Treatment Improvement Protocol
TOPS	Treatment Outcome Prospective Study

Index of Quality Indicators by Topic

Note: This index contains an **alphabetical listing by topic** of the sample quality indicators contained in this report. The indicators were selected as *representative samples* for each dimension. This report is not intended to be a comprehensive compilation of all possible quality indicators relevant to mental health.

Report of the American Psychiatric Association Task Force on Quality Indicators for Children

Approved by the APA Board of Trustees October 2001

Task Force on Quality Indicators for Children

Chair and Editor
James C. MacIntyre, M.D.

Members
Regina Bussing, M.D.
Gabrielle Carlson, M.D.*
Helen L. Egger, M.D.
Emily Harris, M.D.
Joseph Mawhinney, M.D.
Andres Pumariega, M.D.

Consultants
Kelly Kelleher, M.D.
Barbara J. Burns, Ph.D.

Contributors
David Olds, Ph.D.

Staff
Lloyd I. Sederer, M.D.
Deborah Zarin, M.D.*
Claudia Hart
Joyce West, Ph.D., M.P.P.
Farifteh Duffy, Ph.D.
Christine Rose, M.S.*
Cathy Henry, M.P.A.

Liaisons to Other Organizations
Kristin Kroeger
American Academy of Child and Adolescent Psychiatry
John N. Hochheimer, Ph.D.
National Committee on Quality Assurance

Participant through December 1999

Contents

Executive Summary

Charge and Process

In late 1997, the American Psychiatric Association (APA) Task Force on Quality Indicators was established under the chairmanship of John M. Oldham, M.D. The task force was charged with beginning the development of clinically based, patient-focused quality indicators utilizing existing and ongoing research and clinical consensus. The task force completed its work with a final report in March 1999. It recommended the creation of a separate Task Force on Quality Indicators for Children to address the specific issues of children.

Under the auspices of the APA's Council on Quality Improvement, the APA Task Force on Quality Indicators for Children was created in early 1999 with the charge of developing clinically based, patient-focused quality indicators specific to children and adolescents. Members appointed to the task force each brought a different perspective to the effort. Several are active researchers; others have expertise with indicators, accreditation, public/state systems, managed care organizations, and the APA's practice guidelines. Throughout the process, the task force maintained close communication and collaboration with the American Academy of Child and Adolescent Psychiatry (AACAP).

As requested, the task force produced a framework for developing clinically based quality indicators and a set of example indicators specific to psychiatric treatment of children, adolescents, and their families. The *quality framework* was based on a matrix of priority areas and dimensions of treatment. *Recommendations* for each aspect of the framework were also developed. The recommendations address significant concerns in psychiatric treatment and are directed to health facilities, plans, and systems. Each recommendation has one or more examples of *indicators*. Each example of an indicator also includes a proposed *measure* and *standard*. The indicators themselves are exemplars, intended to serve as an initial approach to evaluating mental health care provided to children and adolescents by organized systems of care. The indicators also serve as a source of direction for additional research and development of new indicators.

In presenting its report, the task force emphasizes that the development of quality indicators is a work in progress. The specific examples of indicators given here are not intended to be comprehensive. Many indicators could be substituted to address other important aspects of the broad recommendations about clinical care. Some of the sample indicators are supported by an extensive empirical evidence base; others have more limited research support. Some are more fully developed than others. The degree of practicality and the expense of collecting data required by the indicators vary considerably and are discussed in the full report. The task force encourages others to examine, challenge, or support with research the examples of indicators it is setting forth. It hopes that others will build upon its experience to expand the number of useful indicators in the field of child and adolescent mental health.

The task force has developed this report in a comprehensive and systematic manner. It began by carefully reviewing the March 1999 report of the APA Task Force on Quality Indicators. It also reviewed works in progress by AACAP and other organizations. It established priority concerns and identified relevant recommendations. It defined terms and principles for selection of indicators. And, it solicited advice from consultants and numerous components within APA and AACAP. The process is described more completely in the report, as are the principles that guided selection of indicators.

Definitions

The working definitions used by the task force are as follows:

Recommendation/goal: an important clinical principle that reflects quality patient care

Indicator: a component of quality patient care

Measure: a mechanism or instrument to quantify the indicator

Standard: the level of the measure that suggests that the component of care is of adequate quality (When currently available information does not permit specificity, the level of measure may be used on a comparative basis.)

Quality Framework

The framework developed for identifying and selecting possible quality indicators is as follows:

A. Prevention (access and quality)

1. Universal
2. Selected
3. Indicated
4. Prevention-minded treatment

B. Access

1. Access to appropriate evaluation
2. Access to appropriately qualified clinician
3. Access to appropriate treatment

   a. Psychosocial treatments
   b. Medication
   c. Specialized services

4. Access to continuum of coordinated care
5. Access to culturally and linguistically competent services and providers.

C. Quality/process/appropriateness

1. Comprehensive evaluation
2. Appropriate and effective treatment

   a. Psychosocial treatments
   b. Medication

3. Coordination of services
4. Continuity of care

D. Satisfaction/perceptions of care

1. Patient

   a. Global
   b. Cultural and linguistic competence
   c. Confidentiality

2. Family

   a. Access
   b. Cultural and linguistic competence

    c. Global

    d. Treatment planning

    e. Informed consent

  3. Clinician (provider)

E. Outcomes/effectiveness

  1. Maximization of treatment participation

  2. Reduction or stabilization of symptoms

  3. Improvement in level of functioning of child

  4. Improvement in quality of life for child

  5. Improvement in quality of life for family

  6. Minimization of social and economic costs

  7. Minimization of restrictive care

Workbook of Quality Indicators

Section V, which constitutes the majority of this report, is a workbook of selected quality indicators. This section contains recommendations and goals along with proposed measures and standards for each quality indicator. Discussion and literature references are included for each indicator.

Other APA Efforts

This project complements a range of existing APA efforts. For example, during development of the APA's practice guidelines, potential quality indicators are identified and in some cases operationalized. Diagnosis and assessment projects, such as DSM-IV and the APA *Handbook of Psychiatric Measures,* aim to foster scientifically and clinically appropriate standards. In addition, the APA comments on drafted quality indicators proposed by the government and other quality oversight organizations.

Report Dissemination

The task force believes that its report will be of interest to everyone involved in the child and adolescent mental health services system— those who use and provide services, those who accredit and purchase them, and those who oversee access and delivery. The report will be distributed to appropriate offices and agencies of federal and state government; voluntary accrediting organizations; collegial, medical, and professional associations; consumer advocacy groups; managed care organizations; managed behavioral health organizations; and purchasers. The task force hopes to stimulate dialogue with each of these audiences and to advocate strongly for the delivery of high-quality psychiatric treatment and mental health services to all children and adolescents who require them.

How to Use This Report

The task force acknowledges that the report is lengthy. Efforts have been made to make the report reasonably user-friendly. It is not necessary to read the entire report. Section V (Workbook of Quality Indicators) was designed to provide more detailed information about a limited number of quality indicators. Readers should consider this section as a menu to select a particular dimension (e.g., satisfaction, access, etc.) or individual quality indicators of interest. Readers with a particular topical area of interest can use the appendix to locate specific quality indicators in the report. A standardized format is used to present each indicator. Although somewhat redundant, this presentation enables each indicator to stand on its own and facilitates use by an interested plan, individual, or organization. The *glossary* contains definitions of important terms, and the list of *acronyms* defines acronyms used in the report. The *references* section contains complete citations to all references in the report.

Report of the Task Force on Quality Indicators for Children

I. General Context

A. Trends in the Field

Consumers and purchasers are intensifying their demands for account-ability from the changing health care system, and accrediting and regula-tory organizations are seeking measurable assurances that health facilities, practitioners, and plans are providing quality care. The widespread pro-motion of evidence-based practice guidelines within the field of medicine has coincided with an expanding search for evidence-based indicators that quality care is being delivered and yielding desirable outcomes. De-veloping methods for assessing quality of care has become a priority ac-tivity of government agencies, professional associations, health care plans and facilities, and accrediting organizations (1). This report addresses a missing element in the broad array of indicators that have emerged: qual-ity indicators for mental health services for children and adolescents.

Several factors govern the use of specific quality indicators by health care plans, organizations, and systems: available data sources; the costs and burden of collecting, analyzing, and reporting data; the costs of buy-ing or developing measurement systems; the unique mission or popu-lation being served; and the requirements of accreditation or regulatory organizations. The challenges of collection and analysis of data are dis-cussed with recommendations for specific indicators. The role of account-ability becomes apparent with a review of the activities of national quality oversight organizations.

B. Initiatives of Accrediting or Regulatory Organizations

Quality measures are becoming a standard feature of national health care accreditation programs. Leading organizations include the Joint

Commission on Accreditation of Healthcare Organizations (JCAHO) and the National Committee for Quality Assurance (NCQA).

The **NCQA** issues a Health Plan Report Card, which is intended to help consumers and purchasers compare and select plans that have demonstrated delivery of quality care. Evaluation of each health plan consists of a combination of ratings from an on-site review and the data the plan provides in the Healthplan Employer Data and Information Set (HEDIS). The HEDIS program was developed by NCQA and comprises a set of performance measures that tell how well health plans perform in key areas: quality of care, access to care, and member satisfaction with the health plan and doctors. HEDIS requires health plans to collect data in a standardized way so that comparisons are fair and valid. At present, only a few of the HEDIS measures address psychiatric care, and even fewer address the mental health of children or adolescents.

The predominant focus of **JCAHO** is on hospitals and other health care facilities. The long-range goal of the JCAHO is to accredit health care programs based on an assessment of how well a program complies with JCAHO standards and how well it meets selected performance measures. On December 31, 2000, the JCAHO implemented its requirement that behavioral health care organizations providing 24-hour care with an average daily census of 10 patients or more must select and report quarterly on six performance measures. Because there are no measures required of all facilities to date, the JCAHO is engaged in a major effort to identify standardized *core* performance measures. Core measurement data will be used to monitor a health care organization's performance between triennial on-site surveys and to focus survey evaluation activities.

Although the **American Medical Association** (AMA) has discontinued its program to accredit physicians, it remains committed to determining characteristics and criteria for evaluating physician performance. Hosting the Physician's Consortium on Performance Measurement, the AMA works with experts and representatives of specialty organizations. The consortium is focusing on the development of measures relevant to management of adult diabetes, cardiovascular care, and prenatal testing. Its interspecialty committees are preparing companion documents to assist physicians and their organizations in identifying criteria for selection of physician performance measurement systems.

NCQA, JCAHO, and the AMA collaborate in several venues, which provide a private sector opportunity to develop and coordinate performance measurement activities nationally. This is especially important because each organization emphasizes performance measures for different elements of the health care system (i.e., health care plans, facilities, and physicians).

The **Centers for Medicare and Medicaid Services** (CMS), formerly known as the Health Care Financing Administration (HCFA), provides health insurance for about 75 million Americans through Medicare, Medicaid, and the State Children's Health Insurance Program (S-CHIP). Most enrollees receive their benefits through fee-for-service delivery systems, but a growing number are choosing managed care plans. CMS uses performance measures to help consumers select health care plans that have demonstrated quality care, to set criteria by which plans and providers may be held accountable, and to facilitate quality improvement activities.

Among many initiatives, CMS has mandated the use of performance measure programs in Medicare managed care programs; it is testing them for use in Medicare fee-for-service programs. States have the option of using HEDIS for the Medicaid managed care program. Examples of instruments in use or being piloted include HEDIS, the Consumer Assessment for Health Plans Study (CAHPS), and the Medicare Health Outcomes Survey. In addition, CMS is working with hospital associations, accrediting organizations, and state departments of health to develop and test a standardized core set of hospital performance measures.

The National Forum for Health Care Quality Measurement and Reporting, commonly known as the **National Quality Forum** (NQF), is a not-for-profit organization created in response to a recommendation of the President's Advisory Commission on Consumer Protection and Quality in the Health Care Industry. NQF brings together representation from the public and private sectors. Among other goals, its agenda includes a) development and implementation of a national strategy for measurement and reporting, b) promotion of the collection and dissemination of data needed to improve quality, c) assurance of a systemwide capability to measure and report on quality, and d) standardization programs that will reduce the burden and cost of data collection and analysis to providers and health plans.

The **Institute of Medicine** (IOM) produced a report in March 2001, *Crossing the Quality Chasm: A New Health System for the 21st Century,* emphasizing that America's health system is a fragmented maze that provides excessive and duplicative services while at the same time allowing gaps in necessary care (2). The report calls for coordination of physician groups, hospitals, and health care organizations through a variety of improvements. One is the increased use of technological advances that will allow both caregivers and patients access to key information. The report recommends development of a nationwide technology-based information infrastructure, the identification of common health conditions, and the use of strategies and action plans to improve care for each of these conditions over a five-year period. Implementation will necessitate commonly accepted quality indicators.

II. APA Context

Aware of the national trend to institutionalize data collection and the use of quality indicators, and cognizant of the scarcity of indicators relative to psychiatric care, the APA established the Task Force on Quality Indicators in late 1997. The task force, chaired by John Oldham, M.D., agreed the ideal approach would be to carefully conduct research to determine the most valid and meaningful indicators; however, such work would take several years, large resources, and the cooperation of many disparate facilities and organizations. Consequently, the task force agreed to identify and promote clinically based, patient-focused quality indicators from ongoing research and clinical consensus. The task force completed its work with a final report in March 1999. The report focused on major clinical concerns in mental health and substance abuse care, which were translated into recommendations/goals accompanied by sample indicators, measures, and standards. The report has been disseminated to major accrediting and regulatory organizations. Before completing its work, the task force recommended the creation of a separate Task Force on Quality Indicators for Children to address the specific issues of children and adolescents.

The charge and goals of the Task Force on Quality Indicators for Children are outlined in the next section. Task force members bring different perspectives to the effort. Several are active researchers, whereas others have expertise with indicators, accreditation, state systems, managed care organizations, and the APA's practice guidelines. The task force is chaired by James C. MacIntyre II, M.D. Members include Regina Bussing, M.D., Gabrielle Carlson, M.D., Helen L. Egger, M.D., Emily Harris, M.D., Joseph Mawhinney, M.D. and Andres Pumariega, M.D.

Consultants include Kelly Kelleher, M.D., and Barbara J. Burns, Ph.D. Liaisons were maintained with the APA Council on Children, Adolescents and Their Families, The federal Center for Mental Health Services (CMHS), the NCQA, and the American Academy of Child and Adolescent Psychiatry (AACAP).

Over the life of the task force, many APA staff have participated in this effort: Deborah A. Zarin, M.D; Lloyd I. Sederer, M.D.; Claudia Hart; Joyce West, Ph.D., M.P.P.; Farifteh Duffy, Ph.D.; Christine Rose, M.S; and Cathy Henry, M.P.A.

III. Task Force Approach

A.   Goals of the Project

The task force was charged with the development of a clinically based, patient-focused set of sample quality-of-care indicators as a means to improve the quality of mental health care provided to children and adolescents. This initial set of indicators can be used by APA and other health care groups, including accrediting organizations, as a tool to evaluate the quality of care provided by health plans, providers, managed care organizations, and organized systems of care. The indicators can also serve to improve the quality of care by highlighting important aspects of health care and treatment that need to be addressed by the field, forming the basis for quality improvement research. The work of the task force provides a source of direction for additional research and development of new indicators. The task force will formulate a strategic agenda for APA's role in disseminating quality indicators for children and adolescents.

This project was not intended, nor able, to produce a comprehensive set of indicators. Utilizing the existing evidence base and clinical consensus, the task force developed a limited number of indicators addressing major concerns in the field of child and adolescent mental health and substance abuse care. The report of the Task Force on Quality Indicators for Children will be a "work in progress," undergoing continued refinement and revisions as more data emerge defining the quality of care for children and adolescents. It is the intention of the task force that this report will continue to evolve as a clinically based guide that will be useful to individuals and organizations striving to determine the quality and effectiveness of organized systems of care serving children, adolescents, and their families. The task force expects that current interest in the field will lead to identification of other important and valid indicators.

B. Process

The Task Force on Quality Indicators for Children convened in January 1999 and began its work with a careful review of the final report (March 1999) of the APA Task Force on Quality Indicators (TFQI). In the course of its work, the task force

- Agreed on adoption of definitions, principles, and format contained in the TFQI's final report.
- Examined types of indicators (e.g., structure, process, outcomes).
- Adopted specific definition of terms, such as indicators, measures, standards, priority areas, and dimensions, set forth by the TFQI.
- Discussed whose performance is to be evaluated by indicators advanced by APA.
- Developed a matrix of priority areas and dimensions relevant to quality of mental health care for children and adolescents.
- Developed a set of selected recommendations and goals relating to quality of care in these priority areas and dimensions.
- Developed principles and criteria for selection of specific indicators.
- Developed an initial set of quality indicators corresponding to the selected recommendations.
- Completed a standard information form for each indicator under consideration.
- Sought input from APA committees, the APA Assembly, and the AACAP components regarding the indicators under consideration.
- Consulted with experts in health services research.
- Reviewed proposed indicators for consistency with APA practice guidelines and AACAP's practice parameters.
- Sought support from within the APA to advance the selected indicators for use and/or consideration by external accrediting bodies, government agencies, and others.

The presentation of each indicator includes a title and description, rationale, definition of measure, numerator and denominator, problems or issues in measurement, data quality, potential data sources, potential users and delivery settings, description of standard, and references.

The APA components whose input was solicited included the Assembly; Joint Reference Committee; Council on Quality Improvement; Committee on Quality Indicators; Council on Children, Adolescents, and Their Families; Council on Healthcare Systems and Financing; Council on Psychiatric Services; Council on Research; Committee on Health Services Research; Committee on Standards and Survey Procedures; Committee on Managed Care; and the Committee on Private Practice.

The AACAP components whose input was requested included the Workgroup on Quality Issues, Workgroup on Health Care Reform and Finance, Workgroup on Systems of Care, Workgroup on Training, Psychotherapy Committee, and the Workgroup on Research.

C. Definitions

The task force agreed on the following definitions:

Recommendation/goal: an important clinical principle that reflects quality patient care

Indicator: a component of quality patient care

Measure: a mechanism or instrument to quantify the indicator.

Standard: levels of the measure that suggest the component of care is of adequate quality (When current available Information does not permit specificity, the level of measure may be used on a comparative basis.)

Indicators address various aspects of care and are frequently seen as applicable to structure, process, or outcomes. Indicators that address structure generally look at whether organizational resources and arrangements are in place to deliver quality health care. Indicators that address process, however, examine a series of actions, events, mechanisms, or steps. Outcome indicators, which require the most sophisticated data collection, study the results of a function or process. Outcome indicators may provide the most direct assessment about whether quality care is actually being delivered. Evidence-based process indicators also hold significant promise in assessing quality, since they have been shown to be related to improved outcomes.

When experience and research are available, indicators include thresholds (i.e., standards) that distinguish between acceptable and unacceptable performance. When research is insufficient to support such

benchmarks, this is noted in the report. In the process of operationalizing indicators, it is important to designate whether available data make
it possible to set thresholds or whether comparisons should instead be
made with prior performance or data from similar systems.

The many challenges, complexities, and limitations in applying
available data to the development of quality indicators are widely recognized.

Indicators may measure the performance of an individual provider
or of a hospital or a network of providers in a health care plan. Entire
systems, such as a state mental health system, may also be examined. So
many entities (often interrelated) are involved in providing care that the
task force found itself using the terms *system* and *plan* flexibly. Given its
mandate, the task force selected indicators that depend on aggregate
data—that is, they measure the performance of plans and systems, not
of individual providers.

D. Principles

The task force agreed on the following principles to guide selection of
indicators:

- The indicator addresses an important aspect of care.
- The indicator will be useful in identifying opportunities for improving care.
- The indicator will be practically quantifiable.
- Where possible, the indicator can be documented by evidence-based
  practice guidelines (e.g., AACAP practice parameters, APA practice
  guidelines).
- In areas with insufficient scientific support, expert clinical consensus
  and community standards of practice can be used to support proposed
  indicators.
- The indicator will minimize the potential for unintended adverse consequences.

E. Priority Areas

The task force identified **priority areas** (population categories, psychiatric disorders), some of which were used for the development of the initial set of quality indicators. The selection of priority areas for the initial
indicators was arbitrary, and this report represents a work in progress.

Population categories

- Preschool and school-age children
- Adolescents
- Abused/neglected children and adolescents
- Children and adolescents in special education
- Children and adolescents detained within the juvenile justice system
- Children with severe and persistent mental illness
- Children with chronic medical illness
- Children in child welfare custody
- Families of children and adolescents with psychiatric disorders
- Parents/caregivers with psychiatric disorders

Psychiatric disorders and diagnoses

- Attention-deficit/hyperactivity disorder
- Oppositional defiant disorder
- Conduct disorder
- Depressive disorders
- Substance use disorders
- Psychotic disorders
- Schizophrenia
- Bipolar disorder
- Eating disorder
- Obsessive-compulsive/anxiety disorder
- Axis I psychiatric disorders with coexisting speech/language deficits
- Posttraumatic stress disorder
- Speech and language disorders

F. Dimensions of Treatment

The task force considered **dimensions** of treatment for each of the priority areas. The most useful dimensions are those that can be defined, measured, and improved. After considerable examination and discussion, and on the basis of the work of the former Task Force on Quality Indicators, the Task Force on Quality Indicators for Children decided to give the greatest importance to dimensions of prevention, access, quality, perception of care, and outcome (see Section IV, "Overall Quality Framework").

IV. Overall Quality Framework

Focusing on the priority areas and dimensions noted above, the task force constructed the following **framework** for discussing and selecting possible quality indicators:

A. Prevention (access and quality)

1. Universal
2. Selected
3. Indicated
4. Prevention-minded treatment

B. Access

1. Access to appropriate evaluation
2. Access to appropriately qualified clinicians
3. Access to appropriate treatment

   a. Psychosocial treatment
   b. Medication
   c. Specialized services

4. Access to continuum of coordinated care
5. Access to culturally and linguistically competent services and providers.

C. Quality/process/appropriateness

1. Comprehensive evaluation
2. Appropriate and effective treatment

   a. Psychosocial treatment
   b. Medication

3. Coordination of services
4. Continuity of care

D. Satisfaction/perceptions of care

1. Patient

   a. Global
   b. Cultural and linguistic competence
   c. Confidentiality

2. Family

   a. Access
   b. Cultural and linguistic competence

      c. Global
      d. Treatment planning
      e. Informed consent
  3. Clinician (provider)

E. Outcomes/effectiveness

  1. Maximization of treatment participation
  2. Reduction or stabilization of symptoms
  3. Improvement of level of functioning of child
  4. Improvement of quality of life for child
  5. Improvement of quality of life for family
  6. Minimization of social and economic costs
  7. Minimization of restrictive care

V. Workbook of Quality Indicators

Workbook Format and Organization

The workbook includes a series of quality indicators, measures, and standards that are presented as exemplars for psychiatric treatment of children and adolescents. The specific examples of indicators given here are not intended to be comprehensive. Many indicators could be substituted to address other important aspects of the broad recommendations about clinical care. Some are more fully developed than others. Though some of the indicators are based on a significant amount of research, others have not been scientifically researched. The degree of practicality and the expense of collecting data required by the indicators vary considerably and are discussed in the full report.

    The narrative accompanying each section describes the rationale, need, and importance of the task force recommendations. Also described are the challenges, complexities, and issues raised during development of indicators, measures, and standards for the recommendation/goal. Finally, supporting references and documentation from the literature are provided where available.

Methodological Issues and Practical Considerations

Numerous important methodological and practical issues must be considered in relation to all of the indicators, measures, and standards:

1. *Cultural, linguistic, and ethnic differences:* These indicators, measures, and standards should be utilized with recognition of differences among cultural and ethnic groups. For example, a standard that may be appropriate in one ethnic population may not be in another.

2. *Collection of data—general considerations:* The definition of elements of the measures can be problematic. In many cases, it is difficult to identify individuals with diagnostic or other characteristics from a simple administrative database. In addition, certain evidence or information about types of treatment or relevant outcomes may require more extensive evaluation of medical records, or direct surveys, possibly on a sampling basis.

3. *Collecting/tracking data about parents:* A unique feature of several indicators involves collecting data about parents. This raises issues about the confidentiality of this information and procedural issues regarding the exchange of data between health plans if the parent and child are not enrolled in the same plan.

4. *Collecting/tracking data from other child serving systems:* A unique feature of several indicators involves collecting data from other child serving systems (e.g., schools, juvenile justice system, child welfare/ social services system). This raises issues about the confidentiality of this information and procedural issues regarding the exchange of data between these systems and a health plan.

5. *Confidentiality of data collection and reporting:* Collection of data requires caution about matters of confidentiality. Exchange or collection of patient specific data must also comply with the federal Health Insurance Portability and Accountability Act (HIPAA) regulations in 2002. The task force's selection of indicators has been based on a principle that only aggregate data will be reported; however, some indicators may require an individual chart review to collect relevant information. The task force urges all health systems and plans to develop data collection methods that respect and protect patient confidentiality. Reporting any information that involves identification of an individual patient requires informed consent. Interviews with plan members/enrollees and caregivers (in person or by phone) require informed consent. All written surveys for gathering data should be conducted anonymously.

6. *Designation of standards:* In this report, "standard" is defined as the level of a measure that suggests the component of care is of *adequate* quality. Generally, the designated numerical "standard" represents

an adequate level of performance for a provider or health plan. In some instances, the specific designation of the standard is somewhat arbitrary. Although the overall recommendations derive from evidence-based practice guidelines, the scientific literature, and/or clinical consensus, there may be few data available to translate these recommendations to a population-based standard. Even though strong evidence and universal agreement may exist for a particular recommendation, establishing a standard must take into account that some patients may prefer not to accept particular treatment recommendations. In some cases, patients may have previous experience with treatments that have not been successful. Therefore, it is difficult to determine with accuracy how far below 100% is an acceptable standard. Most standards have been developed in the following manner:

$$\text{Standard } (\%) \ = \ \frac{\text{Numerator (number of individuals meeting the quality indicator)}}{\text{Denominator (total number of individuals in the sample)}}$$

7. *Use of rating scales and standardized instruments:* The report includes references to numerous rating scales and standardized instruments as illustrative examples. The use of such scales and instruments is increasingly supported by APA practice guidelines, AACAP practice parameters, and the emerging evidence base in child and adolescent psychiatry. Many different scales and instruments exist; however, the report does not contain an exhaustive compilation of all that are available. An appendix contains a listing of all the surveys, rating scales, and instruments referenced with specific quality indicators. This appendix may be useful to plans when making decisions about using specific quality indicators and selecting surveys, rating scales, or standardized instruments.

8. *Risk adjustment methodologies:* It is essential that effective methodologies for risk adjustment be developed and applied to the assessment of quality indicators. In many instances, applying the measures included in this workbook might unduly reflect negatively on programs or plans that attract and serve a high proportion of the more severely ill patients or patients with treatment-resistant conditions.

A.   Prevention Indicators

A.1.1.1   **Sample indicator:** Children and adolescents (ages 3–18 years) are screened for emotional and behavioral problems at least annually.

A.2.1.1   **Sample indicator:** Children of adults hospitalized for treatment of affective, anxiety, or substance use disorders or schizophrenia are screened for behavioral disturbances, psychopathology, and functional impairment using an appropriate measure.

A.2.2.1   **Sample indicator:** Adults who are parents and receiving intensive treatment (e.g., inpatient or partial hospitalization) for either affective or substance use disorders also receive appropriate interventions targeting parenting skills.

A.2.3.1   **Sample indicator:** Adults who are parents and receiving treatment for affective, anxiety, or substance use disorders or schizophrenia receive information about the risks, signs, and symptoms of these disorders in children and adolescents.

A.2.4.1   **Sample indicator:** Children enrolled in special education classes/programs are assessed for mental health problems at entry and yearly thereafter with an appropriate assessment instrument.

A.2.4.2   **Sample indicator:** Children in child welfare custody (foster care) are assessed for mental health problems at entry and yearly thereafter with an appropriate assessment instrument.

A.2.4.3   **Sample indicator:** Children with ongoing involvement in the juvenile justice system are assessed for mental health problems at entry and at least annually thereafter with an appropriate assessment instrument.

A.3.1.1   **Sample indicator:** Children and adolescents identified with "sub-syndromal symptoms" of depression, anxiety, or an eating disorder *and* impaired functioning at school receive appropriate preventive intervention.

A.4.1.1   **Sample indicator:** Families of children or adolescents diagnosed with a depressive disorder receive appropriate psychoeducational interventions as part of their treatment.

A. Prevention framework
1. Universal
2. Selected

3. Indicated
4. Prevention-minded treatment

A.1. Specific area: Universal prevention

Universal preventive interventions refer to those interventions that would benefit everyone in the general population or a population subgroup. These interventions are targeted to the general population or a whole population of a specific group but are not identified on the basis of individual risk.

A.1.1   **Recommendation/goal:** The mental health status of children and adolescents should be assessed yearly utilizing a method or measure appropriate for the child's age and development.

The "Bright Futures" initiative focuses on the importance of healthy development in all children and adolescents (3). The federal EPSDT (Early Periodic Screening, Diagnosis and Treatment) program for Medicaid recipients requires periodic screening of health and mental health for children. Assessment should include a developmental history that incorporates an evaluation of mental health development and status (4). For preschool children, identification of oppositional behavior is critical for early intervention. For older children, assessment should cover psychological/psychiatric issues, including anxiety and depression. Information from both the child and an adult (e.g., parent, guardian, teacher) may be necessary.

Age-appropriate questions and/or measures can be used. Interview questions can be used to target issues relevant to a given child or adolescent. Such questions have been included in the recent guidelines for health supervision for infants, children, and adolescents (3), published and available from the National Center for Education in Maternal and Child Health. Standardized measures may also be useful. The Pediatric Symptom Checklist (PSC), a brief psychosocial screening instrument that has been tested broadly in pediatric primary care settings, offers an alternative approach to the recognition of psychosocial problems (5). Inquiring about "parental concerns" is another screening method that can be used (6–7). Older children and adolescents warrant direct assessment. The Patient Problem Questionnaire for Adolescents (PPQ-A) is a self-report instrument used in primary care settings (8). Following the assessment, appropriate referrals should be made to address identified problems and needs.

A.1.1.1   *Sample indicator:* Children and adolescents (ages 3–18 years) are screened for emotional and behavioral problems at least annually.

A.1.1.1   **Sample measure:** Percentage of children and adolescents enrolled in the health plan who receive mental health assessment screening at school or by a physician.

A.1.1.1.1   **Sample standard:** Estimate 85% of children and adolescents will receive mental health assessment screening at school or by a physician.

The numerator proposed for this measure is the number of children and adolescents (ages 3–18 years) enrolled in the plan who receive mental health assessment screening at school or by a physician within the 12-month period. The denominator is the total number of children and adolescents enrolled in the plan during the 12-month period. This indicator presumes that a standardized screening instrument is administered to all enrollees annually. Examples include Pediatric Symptom Checklist (PSC) (5), Columbia Impairment Scale (CIS) (9), Personality Inventory for Children (PIC) (10), Child Behavior Checklist (CBCL) (11–12), and Connors Rating Scales—Revised (13). Data would be collected from a random sample record review (including assessments conducted at school) of patients enrolled in the plan. It is recognized that review of individual records by a health plan is time intensive and may represent a practical limitation for this indicator. As an alternative to record reviews, health plans may use administrative data from their management information system (MIS) if it includes data from the screening instruments. The suggested standard of 85% is based on clinical judgment and may need to be refined.

A.1.1.1.2   **Sample measure:** Percentage of those children and adolescents (ages 3–18 years) who exceed an identified threshold on the screening instrument and are referred for further mental health assessment and evaluation.

A.1.1.1.2   **Sample standard:** Estimate 85% of those children and adolescents encompassed in the measure.

The numerator proposed for this measure is the number of children and adolescents who exceed an identified threshold on the screening instrument and who are referred for further mental health assessment and evaluation. The denominator is the total number of children and adolescents who receive appropriate mental health assessment screening at school or by a physician during the 12-month period. This indicator presumes that a standardized screening instrument is administered to all enrollees annually (see examples listed under A.1.1.1.1). Data would be collected from a random sample record review of patients enrolled in the plan. It is recognized that review of individual records by a health plan is time intensive and may represent a practical limitation for this indicator. As an alternative to record reviews, health plans may use administrative data from their MIS if it includes data from the screening instruments. The suggested standard of 85% is based on clinical judgment and may need to be refined. The "identified threshold" (i.e., scoring on the screening instrument) for determining referral for further mental health assessment would need to be determined by the plan using expert professional consensus and clinical judgment.

A.2. Specific area: Selected prevention

Selective prevention interventions are designed for use with individuals or a subgroup of a population who have a higher than average risk of developing a mental disorder.

A.2.1   **Recommendation/goal:** Children of patients with affective, anxiety, or substance use disorders or schizophrenia should be assessed for evidence of impaired functioning, including school attendance and performance, as well as symptoms of behavior disturbance and psychopathology.

Children of patients with a mental illness are at increased risk for developing a mental illness during their lifetime. Mental illness in a parent(s) places children at increased risk because of genetic vulnerability to a specific illness as well as increased vulnerability to stress (14). Adult patients and families should receive information regarding these increased risks. Children of patients in treatment for a mental illness should be carefully assessed for symptoms of a mental disorder and associated impairment in functioning. Ongoing intervention and treatment, including support for their parents, should be provided to those children who are found to have either symptoms or impaired functioning. Several interventions have been shown to prevent the onset of psychiatric disorders as well as associated morbidity in these at-risk populations. For example, systematic preventive interventions have been developed that target infants and children of parents who are depressed (15–18) and children of parents with substance use disorders (19–21).

A.2.1.1   *Sample indicator:* Children of adults hospitalized for treatment of affective, anxiety, or substance use disorders or schizophrenia are screened for behavioral disturbances, psychopathology, and functional impairment using an appropriate measure.

A.2.1.1   **Sample measure:** The percentage of children with a parent hospitalized for the treatment of a psychiatric disorder (see list above) who receive appropriate mental health assessment screening.

A.2.1.1   **Sample standard:** 85% of the children with a parent hospitalized for the treatment of a psychiatric disorder (see list above) will receive appropriate mental health assessment screening.

The numerator proposed for this measure is the number of children with a parent hospitalized for the treatment of a psychiatric disorder (i.e., affective, anxiety, or substance use disorders or schizophrenia) who receive appropriate mental health assessment screening. The denominator is the total number of children with a parent hospitalized for the treatment of a psychiatric disorder (see list above) during a 12-month period. This indicator presumes that a standardized screening instrument is administered to all children with a parent hospitalized for the treatment of a psychiatric disorder. Examples include Pediatric Symptom Checklist, Columbia Impairment Scale, Personality Inventory for Children, Child Behavior Checklist, and Connors Rating Scales—Revised. Data would be collected from a random sample record review of patients in a 12-month period. It is recognized that review of individual records by a health plan is time intensive and may represent a practical limitation for this indicator. The suggested standard of 85% is based on clinical judgment and may need to be refined.

A.2.2   **Recommendation/goal:** Interventions focused on parenting skills should be provided to those adult patients diagnosed with affective and substance abuse disorders who are involved in parenting.

Parenting can be difficult and stressful for many people. Parenting can be particularly stressful for adults who are recovering from a major mental illness. The level of stress associated with the parenting role can be assessed using the Parenting Stress Index (PSI) (22), and adults receiving intensive treatment for a mental illness should receive assistance with parenting skill development. Examples of preventive interventions that target parenting skills are parenting support groups and structured curricula focused on positive parenting.

A.2.2.1   *Sample indicator:* Adults who are parents and are receiving intensive treatment (e.g., inpatient or partial hospitalization) for either affective or substance abuse disorders also receive appropriate interventions targeting parenting skills.

A.2.2.1   **Sample measure:** The proportion of adults who are parents and being treated intensively for one of the above disorders who are also receiving preventive interventions targeting parenting skills.

A.2.2.1   **Sample standard:** 85% of the adults who are parents and being treated intensively for one of the above disorders will receive the parenting skills intervention.

The numerator proposed for this standard is the number of adults being treated intensively for one of the above disorders who are also receiving preventive interventions targeting parenting skills. The denominator is the total number of adults being treated for one of the above disorders during a 12-month period. Data would be collected from a random sample record review of the adult patients in a 12-month period. It is recognized that review of individual records by a health plan is time intensive and may represent a practical limitation for this indicator. The suggested standard of 85% is based on clinical judgment and may need to be refined.

A.2.3   **Recommendation/goal:** Adults in treatment for depression, bipolar disorder, anxiety disorders, schizophrenia, or substance abuse should receive information regarding the increased risk for development of a mental disorder in children of affected adults. Information about the signs and symptoms that may be associated with the early onset of these disorders in childhood, adolescent, or young adulthood should be included.

Mental illness in parent(s) places children at increased risk for developing a mental illness during their lifetime. In view of this increased risk, parents, along with other family members, spouses, partners, and others in the adult's life, should receive information regarding the risk for mental disorders in children as well as the signs and symptoms that may be associated with the childhood, adolescent, or young adult onset of these mental disorders.

A.2.3.1   *Sample indicator:* Adults who are parents and receiving treatment for affective, anxiety, or substance use disorders or schizophrenia receive information about the risks, signs, and symptoms of these disorders in children and adolescents.

A.2.3.1   **Sample measure:** The proportion of adults who are parents and being treated for one of the above disorders who receive information about the risks, signs, and symptoms of these disorders in children and adolescents.

A.2.3.1   **Sample standard:** Estimate 85% of adults who are parents and being treated for one of the above disorders receive information about the risks, signs, and symptoms of these disorders in children and adolescents.

The numerator proposed for this measure is the number of adults who are parents and being treated for one of the above disorders who received information about the risks, signs, and symptoms of these disorders in children and adolescents. The denominator is the total number of adults being treated for one of the above disorders during a 12-month period. Data would be collected from a random sample record review of the adult patients in a 12-month period. It is recognized that review of individual records by a health plan is time intensive and may represent a practical limitation for this indicator. Health plans would need to identify informational and educational materials for these parents that are appropriate and understandable for the enrolled populations served by the plan. The suggested standard of 85% is based on clinical judgment and may need to be refined.

A.2.4   **Recommendation/goal:** The mental health status of children and adolescents in high-risk subpopulations should be assessed on a regular basis.

Children with chronic medical illness (23–25), children who have experienced child abuse and/or neglect, children with special educational needs (26), children in foster care or residential group homes (27), and children involved with the juvenile justice system (28–29) are at increased risk for mental illness. In view of this increased risk, these children should be carefully assessed for evidence of a mental disorder and impairment in functioning. Health plans should be aware of any enrolled child or adolescent who belongs to one or more of these high-risk subpopulations. Ongoing intervention and treatment, including support for their parents and caregivers, should be provided for those children who are found to have either symptoms or impaired functioning.

Numerous interventions have been developed which target the prevention of psychiatric disorders and associated adverse morbidities such as poor social functioning, out-of-home placement, and high rates of service use. These include interventions for chronically ill children (30–32), young children at risk of abuse and neglect (19–20), children at risk of incarceration (33), and young children at risk of developing aggressive behaviors (34–36).

A.2.4.1   *Sample indicator:* Children enrolled in special education classes/programs are assessed for mental health problems at entry and yearly thereafter with an appropriate assessment instrument.

A.2.4.2   *Sample indicator:* Children in child welfare custody (foster care) are assessed for mental health problems at entry and yearly thereafter with an appropriate assessment instrument.

A.2.4.3   *Sample indicator:* Children with ongoing involvement in the juvenile justice system are assessed for mental health problems at entry and at least annually thereafter with an appropriate assessment instrument.

A.2.4.1.1
A.2.4.2.1
A.2.4.3.1   **Sample measure:** Percentage of children in one of the above circumstances who are assessed for mental health problems with an appropriate assessment instrument at entry and every 12 months thereafter.

A.2.4.1.1
A.2.4.2.1
A.2.4.3.1   **Sample standard:** 85% of children in one of the above circumstances are assessed for mental health problems with an appropriate assessment instrument at entry and every 12 months thereafter.

The numerator proposed for this measure is the number of children and adolescents in the plan who are also in one of the above circumstances and who receive mental health screening with an appropriate assessment instrument within the 12-month period. The denominator is the total number of children and adolescents in one of the above circumstances during the 12-month period. This indicator presumes that a standardized mental health screening assessment instrument is administered at the time of entry into one of the above circumstances (baseline) and annually thereafter. Examples include the Pediatric Symptom Checklist, Columbia Impairment Scale, Personality Inventory for Children, Child Behavior Checklist, and Connors Rating Scales—Revised. The Massachusetts Youth Screening Instrument (MAYSI-2) was developed specifically to screen youths in the juvenile justice system (37–38). Data would be collected from a random sample record review of patients enrolled in the plan. It is recognized that review of individual records by a health plan is time intensive and may represent a practical limitation for this indicator. As an alternative to record reviews, health plans may use administrative data from their MIS if it includes data from the screening instruments. The suggested standard of 85% is based on clinical judgment and may need to be refined.

A.2.4.1.2   **Sample measure:** Percentage of those children and ado-
A.2.4.2.2   lescents who exceed an identified threshold on the screen-
A.2.4.3.2   ing instrument and are referred for further mental health
assessment and evaluation.

A.2.4.1.2   **Sample standard:** Estimate 85% of the children and ado-
A.2.4.2.2   lescents encompassed in the measure.
A.2.4.3.2

The numerator proposed for this measure is the number of children and adolescents in the plan who are also in one of the circumstances above, who exceed an identified threshold on the screening instrument, and who are referred for further mental health assessment and evaluation. The denominator is the total number of children and adolescents in one of the circumstances above who receive appropriate mental health assessment screening during the 12-month period. This indicator presumes that a standardized screening instrument is administered at the time of entry into one of the above circumstances (baseline) and annually thereafter. Data would be collected from a random sample record review of patients enrolled in the plan. It is recognized that review of individual records by a health plan is time intensive and may represent a practical limitation for this indicator. As an alternative to record reviews, health plans may use administrative data from their MIS if it includes data from the screening instruments. The suggested standard of 85% is based on clinical judgment and may need to be refined. The "identified threshold" (i.e., scoring on the screening instrument) for determining referral for further mental health assessment would need to be determined by the plan using expert professional consensus and clinical judgment.

A.3. Specific area: Indicated prevention

Indicated prevention interventions refer to those efforts used with individuals who are at high risk for developing a mental disorder in the future but who currently have minimal signs or symptoms (subclinical or subsyndromal) or the prodromal phase of a disorder.

A.3.1   **Recommendation/goal:** Appropriate preventive interventions should be available for children and adolescents with "subsyndromal symptoms" of depression, anxiety, and eating disorders associated functional impairment.

"Subsyndromal symptoms" refers to those symptoms that incompletely or partially meet the diagnostic criteria defined for a specific mental disorder in DSM-IV-TR. Examples are suicidal ideation in depressive disorders or aggressive behavior in conduct disorder. It is recognized that defining criteria for subsyndromal symptoms is difficult and challenging, given the current state of knowledge and understanding of the evolution of psychiatric disorders.

A.3.1.1   *Sample indicator:* Children and adolescents identified with "subsyndromal symptoms" of depression, anxiety, or an eating disorder *and* impaired functioning at school receive appropriate preventive intervention.

Numerous targeted or indicated preventive interventions have been developed and show utility (39). For at-risk children and adolescents, preventive interventions are available for anxiety disorders (40–41), depression (42–43), conduct disorder (44–46), and eating disorders (47–50). Other examples of preventive interventions include group cognitive intervention for adolescents at risk for depressive disorders (51), intervention with aggressive children at risk for conduct disorder (17, 52), and intervention for children of parents with affective disorder (17).

Most of these interventions include manualized curricula, manualized group interventions, and guided individual intervention programs that can be implemented in naturalistic settings.

Other evidence-based approaches include prenatal and infancy home visiting by nurses (53), parent and teacher education programs about preschool-age children with disruptive behavior problems (54), and violence prevention programs (55–56).

A.3.1.1   **Sample measure:** Proportion of children and adolescents with "subsyndromal symptoms" of a mental disorder (i.e., depression, anxiety, or an eating disorder) and impairment in functioning at school (i.e., poor attendance and/or poor academic performance) who receive appropriate preventive intervention.

A.3.1.1   **Sample standard:** 85% of children and adolescents identified with "subsyndromal symptoms" of a mental disorder (i.e., depression, anxiety or an eating disorder) and impairment in functioning at school (i.e., poor attendance and/or poor academic performance) receive appropriate preventive intervention.

The numerator proposed for this measure is the number of children and adolescents identified with "subsyndromal symptoms" of a mental disorder (i.e., depression, anxiety, or an eating disorder) and impairment in functioning at school (i.e., poor attendance and/or poor academic performance) who receive appropriate preventive intervention (examples listed above). The denominator is the total number of children and adolescents identified with "subsyndromal symptoms" of a mental disorder (i.e., depression, anxiety, or an eating disorder) and impairment in functioning at school (i.e., poor attendance and/or poor academic performance) during a 12-month period.

This indicator presumes that a plan would periodically use a standardized assessment method or instrument to identify children and adolescents who met the criteria for "subsyndromal symptoms." Plans would need to identify specific threshold criteria for the definition of "subsyndromal symptoms" for depression, anxiety, or eating disorder. When a child or adolescent was identified as meeting the criteria, the plan would contact the parent or guardian to get information about school attendance and performance. Plans would also need to identify operational threshold criteria for what constitutes "impaired functioning at school."

Data would be collected from a random sample record review of children and adolescents who met the combination criteria for "sub-syndromal symptoms" and impaired functioning at school during a 12-month period. It is recognized that review of individual records by a health plan is time intensive and may represent a practical limitation for this indicator. The suggested standard of 85% is based on clinical judgment and may need to be refined.

A.4.   Specific area: Prevention-minded treatment

Prevention-minded treatment interventions are designed for those individuals with an identified mental illness who are at severe risk of progression of their mental illness, recurrence, relapse, or developing a co-occurring or comorbid mental disorder.

A.4.1   **Recommendation/goal:** Treatment for all children and adolescents diagnosed with a mental illness should include psychoeducational interventions for the family focused on both the acute illness and recovery.

Family involvement is often mentioned as a critical component of and the context for quality treatment. The AACAP Practice Parameter for the Assessment and Treatment of Children and Adolescents With Depressive Disorders (57) specifically addresses the importance of involving family members as informed partners in the treatment team, helping them understand depression as an illness, addressing psychosocial deficits, and educating them about the importance of compliance with treatment. It is also suggested that participation by parents may help them identify their own depressive symptoms. These are all examples of psychoeducational interventions for families.

A.4.1.1   *Sample indicator:* Families of children or adolescents diagnosed with a depressive disorder receive appropriate psychoeducational interventions as part of their treatment.

A.4.1.1   **Sample measure:** Proportion of families of children or adolescents diagnosed with a depressive disorder who receive psychoeducational interventions as part of treatment.

A.4.1.1   **Sample standard:** 85% of families of children or adolescents diagnosed with a depressive disorder receive psychoeducational interventions as part of treatment.

The numerator proposed for this measure is the number of families with a child or adolescent being treated for a depressive disorder who receive psychoeducational interventions as part of treatment. The denominator is the total number of families with a child or adolescent being treated for a depressive disorder during a 12-month period. Data would be collected from a random sample record review of the child and adolescent patients in a 12-month period. It is recognized that review of individual records by a health plan is time intensive and may represent a practical limitation for this indicator. Health plans would need to develop psychoeducational interventions and materials for parents that are appropriate and understandable for the enrolled populations they serve. The suggested standard of 85% is based on clinical judgment and may need to be refined.

B.   Access Indicators

B.1.1.1   **Sample indicator:** Children and adolescents presenting with symptoms of emotional and behavioral problems receive comprehensive diagnostic and testing services in a timely manner.

B.2.1.1   **Sample indicator:** Health plans have available the full range of licensed mental health professionals who have appropriate training and/or expertise in child and adolescent mental disorders.

B.3a.1.1   **Sample indicator:** Plans provide access to parent training in behavior management of child and adolescent patients diagnosed with oppositional defiant disorder, conduct disorder, or attention-deficit/hyperactivity disorder (ADHD).

B.3b.1.1   **Sample indicator:** Plans provide access to stimulant medication for child or adolescent patients diagnosed with ADHD.

B.3b.1.2   **Sample indicator:** Plans provide access to anti–obsessive-compuslive disorder (OCD) medication for child or adolescent patients diagnosed with OCD.

B.3b.1.3   **Sample indicator:** Plans provide access to antidepressant medication (specifically, selective serotonin reuptake inhibitors [SSRIs]) for adolescent patients diagnosed with major depressive disorder.

B.3c.1.1   **Sample indicator:** Plans provide access to speech and language services for children with speech and language deficits.

B.4.1.1   **Sample indicator:** Children and adolescents with psychiatric disorders have access to appropriate services from a full continuum of care, including emergency services; inpatient, day, and outpatient treatment; crisis intervention; case management; and wrap-around, home-based, and respite services.

B.5.1.1   **Sample indicator:** Plans ensure availability of providers who reflect the ethnicity and language of enrolled populations.

B.5.1.2   **Sample indicator:** Plans provide continuing education programs for their individual providers that focus on culturally and linguistically competent services.

B. Access framework

1. Access to appropriate evaluation
2. Access to appropriately qualified clinicians
3. Access to appropriate treatment

   a. Psychosocial treatment
   b. Medication
   c. Specialized services

4. Access to continuum of coordinated care
5. Access to culturally and linguistically competent services and providers

B.1.   *Specific area: Access to appropriate evaluation*

B.1.1   **Recommendation/goal:** Children and adolescents should have access to and receive appropriate mental health evaluation services.

Appropriate psychiatric evaluation of children and adolescents needs to occur in the context of their developmental status, their social network, and their cultural background. It should result in a diagnostic formulation, an assessment of strengths, and the development of a treatment plan. Pertinent principles have been outlined in the AACAP's Practice Parameters for the Psychiatric Assessment of Children and Adolescents (58–59).

The breadth and intensity of the evaluation need to be determined by providers specializing in child and adolescent disorders and should be tailored to the individual child's needs. The range of required evaluation services may include, but is not restricted to, psychiatric assessments, psychological and psychoeducational testing, speech and language evaluations, laboratory testing, diagnostic imaging, electroencephalograms, and formal development assessments.

Furthermore, *timeliness of care* is a critical component of appropriate access. Standards for timeliness have been developed that distinguish emergency, urgent, and routine care situations. For example, the Children's Special Needs Request for Information (CSNP-RFI) in New York established the following standards for Medicaid recipients (60). For emergency conditions, appointments should be available 24 hours per day, 7 days per week within 1–4 hours. Appointments for urgent care situations, determined through triage not to require immediate care, need to be available within 24 hours. Routine care must be provided within 10 business days. Geographic access standards represent another important domain of access to care. New York's CSNP-RFI (60) also specifies that all enrollees in urban or suburban areas should have access to inpatient as well as outpatient services with 30 minutes travel time or within 30 miles, whichever is less; rural areas may negotiate local standards.

B.1.1.1   *Sample indicator:* Children and adolescents presenting with symptoms of emotional and behavioral problems receive comprehensive diagnostic and testing services in a timely manner.

B.1.1.1   **Sample measure:** Percentage of children and adolescents presenting with symptoms of a psychiatric disorder who receive referral for comprehensive diagnostic and testing services within an appropriate timeframe and geographic distance.

B.1.1.1   **Sample standard:** 90% of children and adolescents presenting with symptoms of a psychiatric disorder receive appropriate evaluation and testing services in a timely manner and within appropriate geographic distance.

The numerator proposed for this measure is the number of children and adolescents presenting with symptoms of a psychiatric disorder receiving appropriate evaluation and testing services in a timely manner and within appropriate geographic distance. The denominator is the total number of children and adolescents presenting with symptoms of a psychiatric disorder. Data would be collected from a random sample record review of patients who presented with symptoms of a psychiatric disorder during the prior 12 months. It is recognized that review of individual records by a health plan is time intensive and may represent a practical limitation for this indicator. The suggested standard of 90% is based on clinical judgment and may need to be refined. The standard is less than 100% because some adolescents and/or parents may prefer not to accept the recommendation for an evaluation.

B.2.   Specific area: Access to appropriately qualified clinicians

B.2.1   **Recommendation/goal:** Children and adolescents should have timely access to appropriately qualified clinicians for psychiatric evaluations, other assessments, and treatment.

The psychiatric evaluation and treatment of children and adolescents differs from that of adults in important respects, requiring additional expertise and training. Evaluation and treatment of children and adolescents requires knowledge of normal and pathological development, as well as familiarity with the range of general medical and psychiatric conditions that affect individuals at different ages. While some mental disorders present similarly across the age spans, others are significantly influenced by developmental factors. As outlined in the AACAP practice parameters (58), competence in developmentally based assessment and treatment principles is essential. Likewise, standardized assessments of children, such as psychological testing, speech and language evaluation, and occupational therapy assessment, require familiarity with age-specific measures and testing principles. An appropriately qualified clinician will have obtained professional specialty training and certification/licensure for child and adolescent populations.

B.2.1.1   *Sample indicator:* Health plans have available the full range of licensed mental health professionals who have appropriate training and/or expertise in child and adolescent mental disorders.

B.2.1.1   **Sample measure:** Percentage of mental health professionals providing evaluation and treatment services to children and adolescents in the plan who have appropriate specialty qualifications and training.

B.2.1.1   **Sample standard:** 90% of mental health professionals providing evaluation and treatment services to children and adolescents have appropriate specialty qualifications and training.

The numerator proposed for this measure is the number of mental
health professionals with documentation of specialty qualifications and
training. The denominator is the number of mental health professionals
providing treatment to this population. Documentation about the qualifications and training of a random sample of individuals providing evaluation and treatment services to children and adolescents during the
prior 12 months would be collected from health plan administrative data.
The suggested standard of 90% is based on clinical judgment and may
need to be refined. The standard is less than 100% in view of the shortage
of child and adolescent specialists in many underserved and rural areas.

B.3.   Specific area: Access to appropriate treatment

B.3a.   Access to appropriate psychosocial interventions

B.3a.1   **Recommendation/goal:** Appropriate psychosocial interventions for the child and family should be available and
used in appropriate intensity and duration for those disorders for which they have been shown to be efficacious,
effective, or clinically indicated.

Recent reviews of research literature on the efficacy and effectiveness of psychosocial treatments for children (61–67) demonstrated durable benefits of psychosocial interventions for a variety of child mental
health disorders. For example, behavioral parent training and behavioral interventions in the classroom are well-established treatments for
ADHD (64). Behavioral management training programs for parents
have been shown to be efficacious for conduct disorder and oppositional defiant disorder. Scientific support is also emerging for other
treatment approaches with these disorders, such as anger management,
assertiveness training, and multisystemic treatment (62). Cognitive-
behavioral interventions have been shown to be probably efficacious
for children and adolescents with depression (63) or with phobias and
anxiety disorders (65). Additional treatment approaches for anxiety disorders based on modeling or operant conditioning principles also have
emerged as probably efficacious. In order to be effective, all interventions should be given in adequate intensity and duration. In addition to

the research evidence, clinical practice reviews and expert consensus opinions have produced additional data.

Evidence and support for using psychosocial interventions are provided in the AACAP practice parameters for depressive disorders (57), bipolar disorder (68), OCD (69), posttraumatic stress disorder (70), other anxiety disorders (71), ADHD (72), conduct disorder (73), substance abuse (74), and schizophrenia (75).

B.3a.1.1   *Sample indicator:* Plans provide access to parent training in behavior management of child and adolescent patients diagnosed with oppositional defiant disorder, conduct disorder, or ADHD.

B.3a.1.1   **Sample measure:** Percentage of children and adolescents diagnosed with oppositional defiant disorder, conduct disorder, or ADHD whose parents received training in behavior management.

B.3a.1.1   **Sample standard:** Estimate parents of 80% of child and adolescents diagnosed with oppositional defiant disorder, conduct disorder, or ADHD receive training in behavior management.

The numerator proposed for this measure is the number of children and adolescents diagnosed with one of the disorders above whose parents received training in behavior management in a given year. The denominator is the total number of children and adolescents diagnosed with one of the disorders above and treated in the plan. Adequate intensity and duration of parent training in behavior management are defined by expert consensus as well as professional practice guidelines and parameters.

Data would be collected from a random sample record review of patients diagnosed with one of the disorders above during the prior 12 months. It is recognized that review of individual records by a health plan is time intensive and may represent a practical limitation for this indicator. Data also might be gathered from the plan's administrative data sets (e.g., claims review data). The suggested standard of 80% is based on clinical judgment and may need to be refined.

B.3b. Access to appropriate medications

B.3b.1   **Recommendation/goal:** Medications, including newer antidepressants and antipsychotics, should be included in the formulary of a given health plan and should be used in appropriate dosage and duration for those disorders for which they have been shown to be efficacious, effective, or clinically indicated.

The safety and efficacy of psychotropic medications for children have been the focus of increasing scientific inquiry. New findings are emerging continuously, necessitating frequent updates of the knowledge and evidence base. A recent review of available evidence on the effectiveness of pediatric psychopharmacotherapy, based on criteria established for the International Psychopharmacology Algorithm Project (76), suggests that the strongest evidence base exists for the short-term pharmacological treatment of ADHD and of OCD (61). The most comprehensively researched treatments for ADHD are the psychostimulant medications (77–79). Further evidence has recently emerged about the efficacy of stimulant treatments for ADHD over a 14-month period (80–81). Efficacious agents for childhood and adolescent OCD include clomipramine (82–84) and SSRIs (85–87). Currently, there is less evidence for the efficacy of SSRI antidepressants for depression. However, support does exist for the use of fluoxetine in the treatment of major depressive disorder in children and adolescents (88).

Additional support and evidence about the use of medications for psychiatric disorders of childhood and adolescence are provided in the AACAP practice parameters for depressive disorders (57), OCD (69), posttraumatic stress disorder (70), other anxiety disorders (71), ADHD (72), conduct disorder (73), bipolar disorder (68), and schizophrenia (75). Psychiatric medications should only be prescribed by physicians who have appropriate experience and training in assessing and treating mental disorders in children and adolescents.

B.3b.1.1   *Sample indicator:* Plans provide access to stimulant medication for child or adolescent patients diagnosed with ADHD.

B.3b.1.2   *Sample indicator:* Plans provide access to anti-OCD medication for child or adolescent patients diagnosed with OCD.

B.3b.1.3   *Sample indicator:* Plans provide access to antidepressant medication (specifically, SSRIs) for adolescent patients diagnosed with major depressive disorder.

B.3b.1   **Sample measure:** Percentage of patients in the health plan diagnosed with the specific disorder who receive a trial of adequate dose and duration of the respective medication.

B.3b.1   **Sample standard:** Estimate 75% of patients with a given disorder receive a trial of the specific medication.

The numerator proposed for this measure is the number of patients diagnosed with the specific disorder who receive a trial of the specific medication in a 12-month period. The denominator is the total number of children diagnosed with the specific disorder in the plan who received treatment for the disorder during the 12 months. Adequate dose and duration are defined by published research, clinical guidelines, or expert consensus publications. Data would be collected from a random sample record review of patients diagnosed with the specific disorder and treated during the prior 12 months. It is recognized that review of individual records by a health plan is time intensive and may represent a practical limitation for this indicator. Data might be gathered from the plan's pharmacy or administrative data sets. The suggested standard of 75% is based on clinical judgment and may need to be refined.

B.3c. Access to appropriate specialized treatment services

B.3c.1   **Recommendation/goal:** Children and adolescents should have access to necessary specialized services for those disorders for which they have been shown to be efficacious, effective, or clinically indicated.

Language, learning, and motor skills disorders affect a large number of children and are frequently associated with other psychiatric and developmental disorders. The assessment and treatment of children affected by these disorders often require multidisciplinary efforts and communication among health professionals and the child's school. Guiding principles have been outlined in several relevant AACAP practice parameters (89–91).

B.3c.1.1   *Sample indicator:* Plans provide access to speech and language services for children with speech and language deficits.

B.3c.1   **Sample measure:** The percentage of children with speech and language deficits who have received or are receiving specialized speech and language services in appropriate intensity and duration and provided by certified speech and language therapists.

B.3c.1   **Sample standard:** Estimate 80% of children with speech and language deficits have received or are receiving speech and language therapy.

The numerator is the number of children who have received or are receiving specialized speech and language services. The denominator is the total number of children identified with speech and language deficits. This will be determined through reviewing treatment plans from a sample of patient records identified by each health plan. It is recognized that review of individual records by a health plan is time intensive and may represent a practical limitation for this indicator. The suggested standard of 80% is based on clinical judgment and may need to be refined.

B.4.   Specific area: Access to a continuum of coordinated care

Since the evolution of the Child and Adolescent Service System Program (CASSP) initiative in the mid-1980s, there has been growing interest in community-based systems of care that offer access to a full continuum of services for children and adolescents with psychiatric disorders. These systems also offer a broad array of alternative or non-traditional services with pooled and/or flexible funding. Development of these programs has been supported by the federal Center for Mental Health Services and the Robert Wood Johnson Foundation. Several recent publications offer support for community-based systems of care. These include *Mental Health: A Report of the U.S. Surgeon General* (92), *Best Principles for Managed Care Medicaid RFPs* (93), and *Best Principles for Managing Outcomes in Managed Medicaid Programs* (94).

B.4.1   **Recommendation/goal:** Interventions of varying levels of intensity and restrictiveness should be available as appropriate for those disorders for which they have been shown to be efficacious, effective, or clinically indicated.

An essential value in serving children and adolescents is provision of service in the least restrictive and most developmentally normative environment. A recent review of effective treatments for children and adolescents distinguishes *traditional forms of treatment* (outpatient therapy, partial hospitalization, and inpatient therapy) from *intensive, comprehensive community-based interventions* (case management, home-based treatment, therapeutic foster care, and therapeutic group homes) and from *crisis support services* (family support, respite services, mentors) (66). These newer approaches have emerged in response to demand for community-based alternatives to traditional services. Presently the evidence base for them lags behind their availability (66). Developmental considerations and family preferences also support the importance of access to a full continuum of care for children and adolescents with psychiatric disorders.

B.4.1.1 *Sample indicator:* Children and adolescents with psychiatric disorders have access to appropriate services from a full continuum of care, including emergency services; inpatient, day, and outpatient treatment; crisis intervention; case management; and wrap-around, home-based, and respite services.

This indicator is not targeted at a specific psychiatric disorder or clinical population. Rather, the indicator is focused on the importance of plan members' having access to a full array of services based on a carefully developed individual plan of care.

B.4.1.1 **Sample measure:** Data will be collected from the plan about the utilization in each service category by enrolled children and adolescents during a 12-month period.

B.4.1.1 **Sample standard:** 100% of plans provide access to a full continuum of services to children and adolescents with psychiatric disorders. A full continuum of services includes emergency services; inpatient, day, and outpatient treatment; crisis services; case management; wrap-around services; home-based services; respite services; and family support services.

Data could be gathered from the plan's administrative data sets (e.g., claims review data). Currently no specific standard has been developed for this indicator. It is anticipated that collecting this data would allow comparison among health plans.

B.5. Specific area: Access to culturally and linguistically competent services and providers

B.5.1 **Recommendation/goal:** Services should be rendered in a manner that is tailored to the cultural and linguistic characteristics of the enrolled population.

Culture and language can serve as barriers to the delivery of appropriate and necessary health services (95–96). Health plans that function in multicultural and diverse linguistic communities should have policies and procedures that support cultural and linguistic competence. Thus, mental health service systems need to identify the health beliefs and practices of enrolled populations to design programs, interventions, and services that will minimize such barriers and ensure cultural competence. Definitions of such efforts have been described in New York's CSNP-RFI (60). Cultural and linguistic sensitivity and competence are among the basic values of the federal CASSP initiative (97).

B.5.1.1   *Sample indicator:* Plans ensure availability of providers who reflect the ethnicity and language of enrolled populations.

B.5.1.1   **Sample measure:** Percentages of providers in the plan who reflect the ethnicity and language of the various enrolled populations.

B.5.1.1   **Sample standard:** Estimate proportional distribution for a given language and ethnicity of plan providers and enrolled patients.

Health plans collect and report data about the language and ethnicity of both children and adolescents receiving treatment and individual providers in the plan during a 12-month period. Data also could be gathered from the plan's administrative data sets (e.g., enrollee demographic data). The suggested standard is based on clinical judgment and may need to be refined.

B.5.1.2   *Sample indicator:* Plans provide continuing education programs for their individual providers that focus on culturally and linguistically competent services.

Continuing education programs must be tailored to the specific cultural and linguistic needs of the plan's enrolled population.

B.5.1.2   **Sample measure:** Percentage of individual providers completing continuing education programs addressing provision of culturally and linguistically competent services to the plan's enrolled population.

B.5.1.2   **Sample standard:** 75% of individual providers have received an appropriate continuing education program within the past 24 months.

The numerator is the number of individual providers in the plan who have received the appropriate training in the provision of culturally and linguistically competent services. The denominator is the total number of individual providers in the plan. Health plans collect and report data about the participation of individual providers in appropriate continuing education programs during the previous 24-month period. Data also could be gathered from the plan's administrative data sets (e.g., provider profiles). The suggested standard of 75% is based on clinical judgment and may need to be refined.

C. Quality/Process/Appropriateness Indicators

C.1.1.1   **Sample indicator:** Children and adolescents receiving treatment for a psychiatric disorder have a multi-axis DSM-IV-TR diagnosis that is based on information that is documented in the evaluation report.

C.2a.1.1   **Sample indicator:** Adolescents diagnosed with depression, OCD, or other anxiety disorders have a trial of cognitive-behavioral therapy (CBT) of appropriate intensity and duration.

C.2a.1.2   **Sample indicator:** Adolescents diagnosed with a depressive disorder have a trial of interpersonal psychotherapy (IPT) of appropriate intensity and duration.

C.2b.1.1   **Sample indicator:** Children diagnosed with ADHD, moderate or severe, receive a stimulant medication trial.

C.2b.1.2   **Sample indicator:** Adolescents diagnosed with a psychotic disorder will receive an atypical antipsychotic medication trial.

C.3.1.1   **Sample indicator:** Children being treated for severe or persistent mental illness requiring multi-system complex care have their care coordinated.

C.4.1.1   **Sample indicator:** Treatment relationships between treating clinician and patient are supported and maintained in the transition between outpatient and inpatient levels of care.

C.4.1.2   **Sample indicator:** If desired by patient and family, treatment relationships between clinician and patient continue to completion of treatment or for a maximum of 6 months under the following circumstances: a) a change in health/

insurance plans or status occurs, or b) the treating clinician leaves the health plan network.

C. Quality/process/appropriateness framework

1. Comprehensive evaluation
2. Appropriate and effective treatment

   a. Psychosocial treatment
   b. Medication

3. Coordination between different levels of care
4. Continuity of care

C.1. Specific area: Comprehensive evaluation

C. 1.1   **Recommendation/goal:** Children or adolescents presenting with symptoms of behavioral, emotional, or learning difficulties need an assessment, sufficiently comprehensive, linguistically and culturally sensitive, and of adequate duration, to establish or rule out the presence of a psychiatric disorder, to make an appropriate DSM-IV-TR diagnosis, and to determine the level of impairment.

The evaluation should include consideration of developmental, medical, neurological, and psychosocial/cultural contributions, following the guidelines for assessment in the practice parameters developed by the AACAP (58–59).

Familiarity with normal childhood development and the principles of child psychiatric diagnosis and treatment is necessary. In addition, essential factors to be considered in assessment, diagnosis, and treatment planning are developmental factors; the roles of caretakers, school, and various social agencies; physical health; and the unique contribution of the family system. Structured or semistructured instruments (98, Table 17–1) can be useful components of the evaluation. However, the evaluation should not depend solely on such instruments. A comprehensive evaluation requires some flexibility in the process, as well as empathic rapport and individualized assessment of feelings, personality style, coping mechanisms, and adaptive strengths. Rating scales and other instruments are also used as part of the assessment and evaluation process. Rating scales are useful in establishing baseline information and to allow ongoing comparison measures (98, Tables 18–1, 19–1, 19–2).

C.1.1.1   *Sample indicator:* Children and adolescents receiving treatment for a psychiatric disorder have a multi-axis DSM-IV-TR diagnosis that is based on information documented in the evaluation report.

C.1.1.1   **Sample measure:** Percentage of children and adolescents receiving treatment who have a DSM-IV-TR diagnosis that is based on evaluation information documented in the record.

C.1.1.1   **Sample standard:** 100% of children and adolescents receiving treatment for psychiatric disorders in the plan have a multi-axis DSM-IV-TR diagnosis which is based on information from their evaluation.

The numerator is the number of children and adolescents receiving treatment who have a multi-axis DSM-IV-TR diagnosis that is based on evaluation information documented in the record. The denominator is the number of children and adolescents who are receiving mental health or substance abuse services. Clinicians may use structured or semistructured instruments in the evaluation process (e.g., Schedule for Affective Disorders and Schizophrenia for School-Age Children [K-SADS], Child Behavior Checklist, NIMH Diagnostic Interview Schedule for Children [DISC]). Data would be collected from a random sample record review of patients who received treatment during the prior 12 months. It is recognized that review of individual records by a health plan is time intensive and may represent a practical limitation for this indicator. The suggested standard of 100% is based on clinical judgment and may need to be refined.

C.2.   *Specific area: Appropriate and effective treatment*

Treatment modalities should be chosen with consideration of therapeutic benefit, risks, linguistic and cultural factors, and patient preference. Appropriate treatment requires ongoing monitoring and evaluation for positive and adverse effects as well as periodic revision of the treatment plan as indicated by response to treatment and additional information. Effective treatment requires an individualized approach based on comprehensive evaluation and the identified patterns of target symptoms and strengths. When evidence and support for specific treatment interventions exists in the literature, these interventions should be provided in appropriate intensity and duration.

C.2a. Psychosocial treatment

Different psychosocial treatments are used to treat psychiatric disorders of children and adolescents. Examples include interactive (play) therapy for children, individual verbal therapy (including psychodynamic psychotherapy), CBT, family therapy, group therapy with peers, and psychoeducational interventions.

C.2a.1   **Recommendation/goal:** Psychosocial treatments should be used in the appropriate intensity, duration, and type for those disorders for which they are likely to be efficacious, effective, or clinically indicated.

Modalities selected should be individualized and based on comprehensive evaluation. Recent reviews of research literature on the efficacy and effectiveness of psychosocial treatments for children (61–67) demonstrated durable benefits of psychosocial interventions for a variety of child mental health disorders. CBT interventions have been shown to be probably efficacious for children and adolescents with depression (63) or with phobias and anxiety disorders (65). Additional treatment approaches for anxiety disorders based on modeling or operant conditioning principles have also emerged as probably efficacious. IPT has also been shown to be efficacious for depression in adolescents (99). Thus, there is increasing evidence that supports the efficacy of using manualized treatments (i.e., CBT and IPT) for depression in adolescents. If a plan provides both CBT and IPT for depressed adolescents, then its estimated that the standard would be 50% of adolescents diagnosed with a depressive disorder receive a course of either CBT or IPT. In order to be effective, all interventions should be given in adequate intensity and duration. In addition to the research evidence, clinical practice reviews and expert consensus opinions have produced additional data. Practice parameters developed by the AACAP contain a synthesis of this data.

C.2a.1.1   *Sample indicator:* Adolescents diagnosed with depression, OCD, or other anxiety disorders have a trial of CBT of appropriate intensity and duration.

C.2a.1.1   **Sample measure:** Percentage of adolescents diagnosed with depression, obsessive compulsive disorder, or other anxiety disorders who receive a trial of cognitive behavioral therapy (CBT).

C.2a.1.1   **Sample standard:** Estimate 50% of patients diagnosed with one of the above disorders receive a course of CBT.

The numerator is the number of adolescents diagnosed with one of the disorders above who received a course of CBT. The denominator is the total number of adolescents diagnosed with one of the disorders above. Adequate intensity and duration of CBT are defined by expert consensus as well as professional practice guidelines and parameters. Data would be collected from a random sample record review of patients who were diagnosed with one of the disorders above during the prior 12 months. It is recognized that review of individual records by a health plan is time intensive and may represent a practical limitation for this indicator. Data also might be gathered from the plan's administrative data sets (e.g., claims review data). The suggested standard of 50% is based on clinical judgment and may need to be refined.

C.2a.1.2   *Sample indicator:* Adolescents diagnosed with a depressive disorder have a trial of IPT of appropriate intensity and duration.

C.2a.1.2   **Sample measure:** Percentage of adolescents diagnosed with a depressive disorder who receive a trial of IPT.

C.2a.1.2   **Sample standard:** Estimate 50% of adolescent patients diagnosed with a depressive disorder receive a course of IPT.

The numerator is the number of adolescents diagnosed with a depressive disorder who received a course of IPT. The denominator is the total number of adolescents diagnosed with a depressive disorder. Adequate intensity and duration of IPT are defined by expert consensus as well as professional practice guidelines and parameters. Data would be collected from a random sample record review of adolescent patients who were diagnosed with a depressive disorder during the prior 12 months. It is recognized that review of individual records by a health plan is time intensive and may represent a practical limitation for this indicator. Data also might be gathered from the plan's administrative data sets (e.g., claims review data). The suggested standard of 50% is based on clinical judgment and may need to be refined.

C.2b. Medication treatment

Psychiatric medication for children and adolescents should be prescribed in both adequate dose and duration in conjunction with psychosocial treatment modalities as clinically indicated.

C.2b.1   **Recommendation/goal:** Medication should be used in treatment of children and adolescents for those disorders for which they have been shown to be efficacious, effective, or clinically indicated.

C.2b.1.1   *Sample indicator:* Children diagnosed with ADHD, moderate or severe, receive a stimulant medication trial.

The safety and efficacy of psychotropic medications for children have been the focus of increasing scientific inquiry. New findings are emerging continuously, necessitating frequent updates of the knowledge and evidence base. A recent review of available evidence on the effectiveness of pediatric psychopharmacotherapy, based on criteria established for the International Psychopharmacology Algorithm Project (76), suggests that the strongest evidence base exists for the short-term pharmacological treatment of ADHD and of OCD (61). The most comprehensively researched treatments for ADHD are the psychostimulant medications (77–79). Further evidence has recently emerged about the efficacy of stimulant treatments for ADHD over a 14-month period (80–81).

The decision to use medication should be based on whether the child or adolescent meets the DSM-IV-TR diagnostic criteria for ADHD and has persistent symptoms that are sufficiently severe to cause functional impairment at school and usually also at home and with peers. Additionally, there should be careful consideration of the risks and benefits of medication, risk of side effects, and outcome or prognosis for the untreated disorder. Medication should not be used as a sole treatment modality. ADHD requires a comprehensive treatment and management plan, which also addresses family, school, and educational needs and symptoms. Coexisting disorders such as specific learning disorders, speech and language disorders, and sensorimotor disorders often require specialized psychotherapeutic or remedial interventions. In most cases, stimulant medication is the first choice of treatment based on the current scientific evidence and expert clinical consensus. Generally, there is a high rate of improvement in both neurocognitive and behavioral symptoms in response to the stimulants. There is some variability in response and dosage among children. The decision to use alternative medications should be based on the following: insufficient clinical response to stimulants; unacceptable side effects or sensitivities; co-occurring conditions that might be aggravated by stimulants; presence of drug-abusing individuals in the home; or prior substance abuse history of the child or adolescent. Alternative medications used in ADHD include antidepressant medications (e.g., tricyclic antidepressants, bupropion, venlafaxine) and adrenergic agonists (clonidine and guanfacine).

C.2b.1.1   **Sample measure:** The percentage of children diagnosed with moderate or severe ADHD who received a trial of adequate dose and duration of stimulant medication.

C.2b.1.1   **Sample standard:** Estimate 75% of patients with moderate or severe ADHD will receive a trial of stimulant medication.

The numerator is the number of children diagnosed with moderate or severe ADHD who received a trial of stimulant medication of adequate dose and duration. The denominator is the number of children in the plan diagnosed with ADHD. Adequate dose and duration are defined by published research, clinical guidelines, or expert consensus publications. Severity of ADHD would be determined by appropriate standardized rating scales or instruments. Data would be collected from a random sample record review of patients who were diagnosed with moderate or severe ADHD during the prior 12 months. An example of a standardized rating scale is the Clinical Global Impressions Scale (CGI). The CGI has been used in ADHD medication studies to assess change. Examples of other scales useful in assessing change and improvement include Connors Teacher Rating Scale—Revised (CTRS-R) and the Connors Parent Rating Scale—Revised (CPRS-R). It is recognized that review of individual records by a health plan is time intensive and may represent a practical limitation for this indicator. The suggested standard of 75% is based on clinical judgment and may need to be refined.

C.2b.1.2   *Sample indicator:* Adolescents diagnosed with a psychotic disorder will receive an atypical antipsychotic medication trial.

There are few controlled studies of the use of antipsychotic medication with children and adolescents who are diagnosed with a psychotic disorder. Case reports and limited research studies indicate effectiveness of both traditional and new generation atypical/novel antipsychotic medications (61). Current clinical practice is guided by expert clinical consensus. Concerns regarding tardive dyskinesia and parkinsonian and dystonic symptoms have diminished use of traditional antipsychotic medications as "first line" choices in favor of the new-generation atypical antipsychotic medications. Clozapine is used for patients with refractory disorder because of its side-effect and risk profile (75). Responsible prescribing requires consideration of both short- and longer-term side effects as well as effects of development. Risk-benefit assessment should also include consideration of the effects of the untreated disorder on both the child and family.

C.2b.1.2   Sample measure: The percentage of adolescents diagnosed with a psychotic disorder who receive a trial of an atypical antipsychotic medication of adequate dose and duration.

C.2b.1.2   Sample standard: Estimate 75% of adolescents diagnosed with a psychotic disorder will receive a trial of an atypical antipsychotic medication.

The numerator is the number of adolescents diagnosed with a psychotic disorder who receive a trial of adequate dose and duration of an atypical antipsychotic medication. The denominator is the total number of adolescents diagnosed with a psychotic disorder. Adequate dose and duration are defined by published research, clinical guidelines, or expert consensus publications. Data would be collected from a random sample record review of patients who were diagnosed with a psychotic disorder during the prior 12 months. It is recognized that review of individual records by a health plan is time intensive and may represent a practical limitation for this indicator. The suggested standard of 75% is based on clinical judgment and may need to be refined. The estimated standard is less than 100% because of the incidence of transient psychotic symptoms that can occur secondary to medication, infectious or metabolic disorders, and illicit/street drugs. The selection of the atypical antipsychotic class of medications is based on the substantial evidence about their efficacy in psychotic disorders with adults. There is, however, currently a lack of evidence regarding the long-term safety and efficacy of using atypical antipsychotic medications with adolescents.

C.3.   Specific area: Coordination of services

Because of the frequent involvement of multiple individuals and multiple systems in the treatment of children, coordination of services and service providers is necessary for appropriate, efficient, and effective care. The specific means or method of providing such coordination should be determined by the treatment team. Coordination of care can be provided in a variety of ways (e.g., a specialized care coordinator or service coordinator; a small team of individuals who share responsibility for coordination). Individuals assigned (e.g., case managers, family care coordinators) should have appropriate training and experience serving children and adolescents across multiple systems of care (e.g., mental health, school, child welfare, juvenile justice). These individuals who are coordinating care should also have demonstrated cultural and linguistic competence.

C.3.1   **Recommendation/goal:** Children with severe or persistent mental illness whose care involves multiple child serving systems, caretakers, and service providers should have their care coordinated.

C.3.1.1   *Sample indicator:* Children being treated for severe or persistent mental illness requiring multisystem complex care have their care coordinated.

C.3.1.1   **Sample measure:** The percentage of children with severe or persistent mental illness are either assigned an individual to provide coordination (e.g., case manager, care coordinator) or have evidence of coordination of services.

C.3.1.1   **Sample standard:** Estimate 80% of children being treated for severe or persistent mental illness will have evidence of coordination of care.

The numerator is the number of children with severe or persistent mental illness who were either assigned a case manager/coordinator or whose case demonstrates evidence of coordinated services. The denominator is the total number of children impaired because of severe and persistent mental illness who received treatment in the plan. Plans would need to develop definitions of "severe or persistent mental illness" and "evidence." Data would be collected from a random sample record review of patients who were admitted and diagnosed with severe or recurrent mental illnesses during the prior 12 months. It is recognized that review of individual records by a health plan is time intensive and may represent a practical limitation for this indicator. The suggested standard of 80% is based on clinical judgment and may need to be refined.

C.4. Specific area: Continuity of care

Continuity of care supports effective treatment through the therapeutic alliance, continuing awareness of past treatment experience and history, and prevention of interruption and/or fragmentation of treatment. Studies of patients who drop out of treatment indicate that lack of continuity is an important source of patient dissatisfaction with treatment (100).

C.4.1   **Recommendation/goal:** Continuity of the treatment relationship should be supported and maintained through both level of care transitions and change of insurance plans for up to 6 months or until terminated due to resolution of illness or at patient's family request.

C.4.1.1   *Sample indicator:* Treatment relationships between clinician and patient are supported and maintained in the transition between outpatient and inpatient levels of care.

Outpatient clinicians may be involved with the inpatient episode of care in various ways. Examples include exchanging written information, telephone calls, and/or actual face-to-face meetings. This does not necessarily mean, however, that the outpatient clinician would be the primary clinician for the child's inpatient admission.

C.4.1.1   **Sample measure:** The percentage of outpatient clinicians who continue some contact or involvement with the patient and/or treatment team when he or she is admitted to inpatient care.

C.4.1.1   **Sample standard:** Estimated 75% of outpatient clinicians maintain some involvement with their patient and/or treatment team during inpatient care.

The numerator is the number of children and adolescents whose outpatient therapists maintained some involvement during their inpatient psychiatric admission. The denominator is all children and adolescents who had an inpatient admission. Data about the therapist's involvement would be collected from a random sample record review of patients who had an inpatient psychiatry admission during the prior 12 months. It is recognized that review of individual records by a health plan is time intensive and may represent a practical limitation for this indicator. The suggested standard of 75% is based on clinical judgment and may need to be refined.

C.4.1.2   *Sample indicator:* If desired by patient and family, treatment relationships between clinician and patient continue to completion of treatment or for a maximum of 6 months under the following circumstances: a) a change in health/insurance plans or status occurs or b) the treating clinician leaves the health plan network.

The NCQA encourages continued access to a clinician who is leaving a plan network. The NCQA standard for managed care organizations (2001–2002) indicates that plan members undergoing active treatment should have access to their practitioner through the current period of active treatment or for up to 90 days, whichever is shorter (101). Plans should strive to attract and retain high-quality providers of mental health services. Retention rates of quality providers can be used to compare health plans.

C.4.1.2   **Sample measure:** Percentage of clinician/patient treatment relationships that continue, when desired by patient and family, to completion of treatment or for a maximum of 6 months under the two circumstances listed above.

C.4.1.2   **Sample standard:** Estimated 75% of treatment relationships continuing when desired by the patient and family under the circumstances listed above.

The numerator is the number who continue treatment (to completion or up to a maximum of 6 months) with the same clinician under the circumstances listed above. The denominator is the total number of children in the circumstances listed above whose families desired continuing treatment with the same clinician. Data would be collected from a sample record review of patients in the two categories: a) those who left the health plan during the prior 12 months and b) those whose treating clinician left the health plan's network. It is recognized that review of individual records by a health plan is time intensive and may represent a practical limitation for this indicator. The suggested standard of 75% is based on clinical judgment and may need to be refined. The recommendation of "to completion of treatment or for a maximum of 6 months" is also based on clinical judgment.

D.   Satisfaction/Perceptions of Care Indicators

D.1a.1.1   **Sample indicator:** Adolescent members using mental health or substance abuse services are either very or highly satisfied.

D.1b.1.1   **Sample indicator:** Adolescent members using mental health or substance abuse services are either very or highly satisfied with the cultural and linguistic competence of these services.

D.1c.1.1   **Sample indicator:** Adolescent members using mental health or substance abuse services are either very or highly satisfied with the confidentiality of these services.

D.2a.1.1   **Sample indicator:** Families of child or adolescent members are either very or highly satisfied with access to mental health or substance abuse services.

D.2b.1.1   **Sample indicator:** Families with a child or adolescent using mental health or substance abuse services are either very or highly satisfied with the cultural and linguistic competence of these services.

D.2c.1.1   **Sample indicator:** Families of child or adolescent members using mental health or substance abuse services are satisfied with their treatment services.

D.2d.1.1   **Sample indicator:** Families with a child or adolescent using mental health or substance abuse services are either very or highly satisfied with their involvement in treatment planning for their child.

D.2e.1.1   **Sample indicator:** Families with a child or adolescent using mental health or substance abuse services are satisfied with the discussion of treatment options and risks and benefits.

D.3.1.1   **Sample indicator:** Network providers of mental health or substance abuse services are either very or highly satisfied with the behavioral health plan.

D. Satisfaction/perceptions of care framework

1. Patient
   a. Global
   b. Cultural and linguistic competence
   c. Confidentiality

   2. Family
      a. Access
      b. Cultural and linguistic competence
      c. Global
      d. Treatment planning
      e. Informed consent
   3. Clinician (provider)

   Consumer satisfaction is an important measure of the quality of behavioral health care and is crucial in the evaluation of outpatient mental health services. It is viewed as an important sentinel of potential problems in health care delivery. Satisfaction is linked to health care, treatment compliance, health status outcome, and changes in one's doctor or health plan (102–106). Satisfaction may be measured along several dimensions. These include the method used to contact respondents (mail, interview, telephone), the target (visit, provider, clinic, plan), and the domain. Domains of consumer satisfaction include perceived quality of care provided; perceptions of the care experience; outcomes of care; and interpersonal factors with regard to the way care is provided.

   Patient satisfaction ratings reflect perceptions and assumptions about health care and the way it should be provided. In the future, reports of patient satisfaction will assume greater weight in the awarding of managed care contracts than they have in the past (105). There is increasing recognition that an evaluation of managed care should examine how mental health services impact children with chronic conditions such as mental disorders. Specific efforts include reporting HEDIS quality and satisfaction measures separately for these populations (107). Dissatisfaction with one's health plan may lead to plan disenrollment and out-of-plan use (108–110); general satisfaction with care has effects on patient compliance with treatment plans and choice of physicians (109, 111).

   The general practice among health plans and health services researchers is to survey the insured party (i.e., the parent) about issues of satisfaction for all family members. Most previous attempts to improve the quality of care for adolescents have examined the perceptions and satisfaction levels of their parents (112–116). This strategy works for younger children but is much less reliable for older children. Parents are more likely to make and enforce decisions about treatment for their younger children, whereas parents have less control of their adolescents' attitudes and attendance. Therefore, when the perspectives of adolescents are not taken into account, the evaluation of services is theoretically incomplete and biased toward the views of parents, provider, and/or evaluator (117–120). Satisfaction at the health plan level is usually assessed through mailed or telephone surveys. Instruments administered at the clinic level are not ideal because they do not capture results from persons who drop out of care, do not come to appointments, or lack access. The use of mail surveys with reminders is standard practice for adults in commercial plans but has not been successful in Medicaid plans or with adolescents. Thus, telephone surveys, which are expensive, will be required for these efforts. Finally, provider surveys require telephone surveys for the most part.

This section addresses overall plan satisfaction issues from various informants. Eventually, separate reporting and assessment procedures should be developed for "priority populations," such as children in substitute care, the severely disturbed, and minority populations, since prior work has demonstrated the needs for different instruments, reporting methods, and results.

D.1. Specific area: Patient satisfaction

D.1a. Adolescent member global satisfaction

Adolescents report more satisfaction with individual treatment and less satisfaction with family therapy, whereas parents report more satisfaction with family therapy and less satisfaction with individual treatment for their children (113). Adolescents' satisfaction is actually linked to both the structural and interpersonal therapeutic aspects of service delivery. Their attitude before the actual visit and their perceptions of a provider's performance, as well as the waiting time to see the provider, are important to how they rate satisfaction. Their degree of satisfaction is as much a reflection of their own psychosocial characteristics as it is of the actual care they receive (106, 121–122). Their satisfaction with services is a reliable predictor of their subsequent compliance with appointments, intention to return, or follow-up. Factors that are important to adolescents include confidentiality, respect for privacy, characteristics of the provider, frequency and duration of services, scheduling, enjoyability, accessibility, and the provider's explanation of the rationale for treatment, interventions, and outcome (105).

D.1a.1   **Recommendation/goal:** A high proportion of children and adolescents using behavioral services should be very satisfied with their services.

D.1a.1.1   *Sample indicator:* Adolescent members using mental health or substance abuse services are either very or highly satisfied.

D.1a.1.1   **Sample measure:** With use of a standardized instrument, the percentage of adolescents using mental health or substance abuse services in a given year who report being either very or highly satisfied with those services.

D.1a.1.1   **Sample standard:** Estimate 65% of adolescent patients using mental health or substance abuse services will report being either very or highly satisfied with those services.

The numerator proposed for this measure is the number of adolescent patients using mental health or substance abuse services who report on a standardized instrument that they are either very or highly satisfied with their behavioral health services. The denominator is the total number of adolescents receiving mental health or substance abuse services in the plan during a 12-month period. This indicator presumes that a standardized instrument is used at intervals during the course of treatment. One example is the Consumer Assessment of Behavioral Health Services (CABHS) (123–124). Data would be collected from a random sample record review of patients receiving mental health or substance abuse services in the plan during a 12-month period. It is recognized that review of individual records by a health plan is time intensive and may represent a practical limitation for this indicator. As an alternative to record reviews, health plans may use administrative data from their MIS if it includes data from the rating instruments. The suggested standard of 65% is based on clinical judgment and may need to be refined.

D.1b. Adolescent satisfaction with cultural and linguistic competence of behavioral health services

The rapid growth of minority populations in the United States and the recognition that cultural and linguistic barriers to mental health services present formidable obstacles to mental health care require attention to the cultural competence of behavioral health services. To date, there is a dearth of adolescent or family assessment surveys about cultural competence. However, some new measures exist that may be relevant (125).

D.1b.1   **Recommendation/goal:** A high proportion of adolescents using behavioral health services should be very satisfied with the cultural and linguistic competence of their care.

D.1b.1.1   *Sample indicator:* Adolescent members using mental health or substance abuse services are either very or highly satisfied with the cultural and linguistic competence of these services.

D.1b.1.1   **Sample measure:** Using a standardized instrument, the percentage of adolescent patients using mental health or substance abuse services in a given year who report being either very or highly satisfied with the cultural and linguistic competence of behavioral services.

D.1b.1.1   **Sample standard:** Estimate 65% of adolescent patients will report being very or highly satisfied with the cultural and linguistic competence of their behavioral services.

The numerator proposed for this measure is the number of adolescent patients using mental health or substance abuse services who report on a standardized instrument that they are either very or highly satisfied with the cultural and linguistic competence of their behavioral health services. The denominator is the total number of adolescents receiving mental health or substance abuse services in the plan during a 12-month period. This indicator presumes that a standardized instrument is used at intervals during the course of treatment. Examples include Consumer Assessment of Behavioral Health Services (123–124), Tools for Monitoring Cultural Competence (126), and Cross Cultural Counseling Inventory (CCCI-R) (127). Data would be collected from a random sample record review of patients receiving mental health or substance abuse services in the plan. It is recognized that review of individual records by a health plan is time intensive and may represent a practical limitation for this indicator. As an alternative to record reviews, health plans may use administrative data from their MIS if it includes data from the rating instruments. The suggested standard of 65% is based on clinical judgment and may need to be refined.

D.1c. Adolescent member satisfaction with confidentiality of behavioral services

Adolescent concerns about confidentiality have been labeled as some of the most important barriers to behavioral health care access. Adolescents in particular may be susceptible to concerns about parent awareness of their emotional and behavioral symptoms. Thus, confidentiality around their behavioral concerns is particularly important.

D.1c.1   **Recommendation/goal:** A high proportion of adolescents using behavioral health services should be very satisfied with the confidentiality of their care.

D.1c.1.1   *Sample indicator:* Adolescent members using mental health or substance abuse services are either very or highly satisfied with the confidentiality of these services.

D.1c.1.1   **Sample measure:** Using a standardized instrument, the proportion of adolescent patients using mental health or substance abuse services who report being very or highly satisfied with confidentiality of behavioral health services.

D.1c.1.1   **Sample standard:** 85% of adolescent patients using mental health or substance abuse services will report being either very or highly satisfied with the confidentiality of their behavioral health services.

The numerator proposed for this measure is the number of adolescent patients using mental health or substance abuse services who report on a standardized instrument that they are either very or highly satisfied with the confidentiality of their behavioral health services. The denominator is the total number of adolescents receiving mental health or substance abuse services in the plan during a 12-month period. This indicator presumes that a standardized instrument is used at intervals during the course of treatment. An example is the Consumer Assessment of Behavioral Health Services (123–124). Data would be collected from a random sample record review of patients receiving mental health or substance abuse services in the plan. It is recognized that review of individual records by a health plan is time intensive and may represent a practical limitation for this indicator. As an alternative to record reviews, health plans may use administrative data from their MIS if it includes data from the rating instruments. The suggested standard of 85% is based on clinical judgment and may need to be refined.

D.2.   Specific area: Family satisfaction

Parental satisfaction is linked to structural and economic aspects of children's services. Parents are more likely to base their satisfaction on access and convenience, their child's treatment process (including the relationship with the therapist), availability of parent and family services, and overall ease of the process. They are more satisfied with services when parents and providers mutually agree to terminate a child's outpatient treatment services. And, the longer the child is in treatment, the more satisfied parents are with their relationship with the child's therapist (105, 116). Stuntzer-Gibson et al. describe the factors affecting older children's perspectives on service satisfaction (128): "Older children possess greater critical awareness and cognitive ability to evaluate events in their lives. They may expect more of services and consequently derive less satisfaction from them. In addition, older children generally have more complex needs owing to their maturational development, and services may not be sufficiently attuned to these needs. Thus their dissatisfaction may be as much a reflection of service systems inadequacies as it is higher critical standards."

D.2a. Family members' satisfaction with access to behavioral services

D.2a.1   **Recommendation/goal:** A high proportion of families with children should be aware of how to access behavioral health services and satisfied with their access to services.

D.2a.1.1   *Sample indicator:* Families of child or adolescent members are either very or highly satisfied with access to mental health or substance abuse services.

D.2a.1.1   **Sample measure:** Using appropriate standardized measures, the percentage of families with a child or adolescent who report satisfaction with access to mental health or substance abuse services—including choice of providers, ease in obtaining appointments and referrals, and paperwork burden.

D.2a.1.1.1   **Sample standard:** Estimate 85% of families with a child or adolescent receiving treatment will be satisfied with their access to mental health and substance abuse services.

The numerator proposed for this measure is the number of families among those responding who report being either very or highly satisfied with their access to mental health or substance abuse services on a standardized instrument. The denominator is the total number of families enrolled in the plan during a 12-month period. This indicator presumes that a standardized instrument or survey is used at intervals to collect information. Examples include Consumer Assessment of Behavioral Health Services (123–124) and Parent Assessment of Care Survey (PACS) (129). Data could also be collected from caregiver interviews using a random sample of families enrolled in the plan. It is recognized that caregiver interviews by a health plan are time intensive and may represent a practical limitation for this indicator. As an alternative to caregiver interviews, health plans may use administrative data from their MIS if it includes data from the standardized instrument. The suggested standard of 85% is based on clinical judgment and may need to be refined.

D.2b. Family members' satisfaction with cultural and linguistic competence

D.2b.1   **Recommendation/goal:** A high proportion of families with children should be satisfied with the cultural and linguistic competence of their behavioral health services.

The rapid growth of minority populations in the United States and the recognition that cultural and linguistic barriers present formidable obstacles to mental health care require attention. To date, there is a dearth of adolescent or family assessment surveys of cultural competence. However, some new measures exist that may be relevant (125).

D.2b.1.1   *Sample indicator:* Families with a child or adolescent using mental health or substance abuse services are either very or highly satisfied with the cultural and linguistic competence of these services.

D.2b.1.1   **Sample measure:** The proportion of families with a child or adolescent using mental health or substance abuse services who report, through use of a standardized instrument, being very or highly satisfied with the cultural and linguistic competence of services.

D.2b.1.1   **Sample standard:** 85% of families with a child or adolescent using mental health of substance abuse services report being either very or highly satisfied with cultural and linguistic competence of mental health or substance abuse services.

The numerator proposed for this measure is the number of families with a child or adolescent using mental health or substance abuse services who report on a standardized instrument that they are either very or highly satisfied with the cultural and linguistic competence of the services. The denominator is the total number of families with a child or adolescent receiving mental health or substance abuse services in the plan during a 12-month period. This indicator presumes that a standardized instrument is used at intervals during the course of treatment. Examples include Consumer Assessment of Behavioral Health Services (123–124), Tools for Monitoring Cultural Competence (126), Cross Cultural Counseling Inventory (127), and Parent Assessment of Care Survey (129). Data would be collected from a random sample record review of patients receiving mental health or substance abuse services in the plan. It is recognized that review of individual records by a health plan is time intensive and may represent a practical limitation for this indicator. As an alternative to record reviews, health plans may use administrative data from their MIS if it includes data from the rating instruments. The suggested standard of 85% is based on clinical judgment and may need to be refined.

D.2c. Family members' global satisfaction

D.2c.1   **Recommendation/goal:** A high proportion of families with children should be satisfied with their behavioral health treatment services.

D.2c.1.1   *Sample indicator:* Families of child or adolescent members using mental health or substance abuse services are satisfied with their treatment services.

D.2c.1.1   **Sample measure:** The proportion of families with a child or adolescent using mental health or substance abuse services who report, through of a standardized instrument, being satisfied with these treatment services.

D.2c.1.1   **Sample standard:** 85% of families with a child or adolescent using mental health or substance abuse services report being satisfied with these treatment services.

The numerator proposed for this measure is the number of families with a child or adolescent using mental health or substance abuse services who report on a standardized instrument that they are satisfied with the treatment services. The denominator is the total number of families with a child or adolescent receiving mental health or substance abuse services in the plan during a 12-month period. This indicator presumes that a standardized instrument is used at intervals during the course of treatment. Examples include Consumer Assessment of Behavioral Health Services (123–124) and Parent Assessment of Care Survey (129). Data would be collected from a random sample record review of patients receiving mental health or substance abuse services in the plan. It is recognized that review of individual records by a health plan is time intensive and may represent a practical limitation for this indicator. As an alternative to record reviews, health plans may use administrative data from their MIS if it includes data from the rating instruments. Data could also be collected from caregiver interviews using a random sample of families receiving mental health or substance abuse services. It is recognized that caregiver interviews conducted by a health plan are time intensive and may represent a practical limitation for this indicator. The suggested standard of 85% is based on clinical judgment and may need to be refined.

D.2d. Parental/guardian satisfaction with involvement in treatment planning

D.2d.1   **Recommendation/goal:** Health plans should systematically and regularly assess parent/guardian satisfaction with the degree to which they are included in treatment planning for their child and planning for crisis or emergency management.

D.2d.1.1   *Sample indicator:* Families with a child or adolescent using mental health or substance abuse services are either very or highly satisfied with their involvement in treatment planning for their child.

D.2d.1.1   **Sample measure:** The proportion of families with a child or adolescent using mental health or substance abuse services who report, through use of a survey instrument, that they are either very or highly satisfied with their involvement in treatment planning.

D.2d.1.1   **Sample standard:** Estimate 85% of families with a child or adolescent using mental health or substance abuse services will report that they are either very or highly satisfied with their involvement in treatment planning.

NOTE: To determine their involvement, the parents or caregivers are asked if they feel that their role in their child's care was acknowledged by staff and if they had the opportunity to participate in treatment planning and planning for management of crises and emergencies.

The numerator proposed for this measure is the number of families with a child or adolescent using mental health and substance abuse services who report that they are either very or highly satisfied with their involvement in treatment planning. The denominator is the total number of families with a child or adolescent receiving mental health or substance abuse services during a 12-month period. This indicator presumes that a survey is used at intervals to collect information. Data could also be collected from caregiver interviews using a random sample of families. It is recognized that caregiver interviews by a health plan are time intensive and may represent a practical limitation for this indicator. As an alternative to caregiver interviews, health plans may use administrative data from their MIS if it includes data from the survey instrument. The suggested standard of 85% is based on clinical judgment and may need to be refined.

D.2e. Parent/guardian satisfaction with informed consent process

This specifically refers to satisfaction with the provider's discussion of treatment options/treatment risks and benefits and how he or she obtained informed consent/assent for treatment.

D.2e.1   **Recommendation/goal:** Health plans should systematically and regularly assess parent/guardian satisfaction with the way the provider discussed treatment options/treatment risks and benefits and obtained informed consent from the parent and informed assent from the child.

D.2e.1.1   *Sample indicator:* Families with a child or adolescent using mental health or substance abuse services are satisfied with the discussion of treatment options, risks, and benefits.

D.2e.1.1   **Sample measure:** The proportion of families with a child or adolescent using mental health or substance abuse services who report, through use of a survey instrument, that they are satisfied with the discussion of treatment options, risks, and benefits by the treatment provider(s).

D.2e.1.1   **Sample standard:** Estimate 85% of families with a child or adolescent using mental health or substance abuse services who report that they are satisfied with the discussion of treatment options, risks, and benefits by the treatment provider(s).

The numerator proposed for this measure is the number of families with a child or adolescent using mental health and substance abuse services who report that they are satisfied with the discussion of treatment options, risks, and benefits. The denominator is the total number of families with a child or adolescent receiving mental health or substance abuse services during a 12-month period. This indicator presumes that a survey instrument is used at intervals to collect information. The survey should assess a) parental satisfaction with the quantity and quality of information received from the clinician about treatment benefits and risks and treatment options, and b) whether informed consent was obtained from the parents and informed assent from the child.

Data could also be collected from caregiver interviews using a random sample of families. It is recognized that caregiver interviews by a health plan are time intensive and may represent a practical limitation for this indicator. As an alternative to caregiver interviews, health plans may use administrative data from their MIS if it includes data from the survey. The suggested standard of 85% is based on clinical judgment and may need to be refined.

D.3. Specific area: Clinician/provider satisfaction

Increasingly it is apparent that clinician/provider satisfaction with a health plan can affect access of enrolled members to clinician/providers.

D.3.1   **Recommendation/goal:** A high proportion of network providers should be satisfied with administrative services, values, and quality of care and with their ability to choose and implement treatments provided through the behavioral health plan.

D.3.1.1   *Sample indicator:* Network providers of mental health or substance abuse services are either very or highly satisfied with the behavioral health plan.

D.3.1.1   **Sample measure:** The percentage of network providers who report, through use of a survey instrument, they are highly or very satisfied with a) the plan's administrative services, values, and quality of care; and b) the provider's ability to choose and implement behavioral health treatments provided through the plan.

D.3.1.1   **Sample standard:** Estimate 70% of network providers will be satisfied overall.

The numerator proposed for this measure is the number of network providers of mental health or substance abuse services who report that they are satisfied with the plan's administrative services, values, and quality of care. The denominator is the total number of network providers of mental health or substance abuse services to children and adolescents during a 12-month period. This indicator presumes that a survey instrument is used at intervals to collect information. The survey should assess a) satisfaction with the plan's administrative services, values, and quality of care, and b) the provider's ability to choose and implement behavioral treatments provided through the plan.

Data could also be collected by interviewing a random sample of network providers. It is recognized that network provider interviews conducted by a health plan are time intensive and may represent a practical limitation for this indicator. The suggested standard of 70% is based on clinical judgment and may need to be refined. In lieu of using a fixed percentage as the standard, plans could choose to demonstrate continuous improvement in network provider satisfaction with the plan.

E.   Outcomes/Effectiveness Indicators

E.1.1.1   **Sample indicator:** Children and families participate in the decision to terminate treatment in a health plan.

E.2.1.1   **Sample indicator:** Reduction in symptoms of inattention, impulsivity, and hyperactivity among patients with the diagnosis of ADHD receiving treatment for the disorder in a given health plan.

E.2.1.2   **Sample indicator:** Reduced use of substances among patients with a diagnosis of a substance-related disorder (abuse or dependence) who are receiving treatment for the disorder in a given health plan.

E.3.1.1   **Sample indicator:** Improved school attendance for children and adolescents receiving treatment for a psychiatric disorder in a given health plan.

E.3.1.2   **Sample indicator:** Decreased involvement (i.e., arrests, detentions, or incarcerations) with juvenile justice/criminal system for children and adolescents receiving treatment for a psychiatric disorder in a health plan.

E.3.1.3   **Sample indicator:** Children and adolescents diagnosed with a psychotic disorder receiving treatment for the disorder will demonstrate an improved level of functioning.

E.4.1.1   **Sample indicator:** Children and adolescents receiving treatment for a mental disorder report increased enjoyment of life and fuller participation in age and/or developmentally appropriate activities.

E.4.2.1   **Sample indicator:** Absence of documented abuse or neglect subsequent to the initiation of treatment of children in a given health plan.

E.5.1.1   **Sample indicator:** Reduction in family's stress level and impact of illness.

E.6.1.1   **Sample indicator:** Plans strive to limit the number of days of work missed by parents due to caring for a child receiving treatment for a mental disorder in a given health plan.

E.6.1.2   **Sample indicator:** Plans strive to limit the number of days of homebound instruction for children receiving treatment for a mental disorder in a given health plan.

E.7.1.1   **Sample indicator:** Plans strive to limit the number of days children receiving treatment for a mental disorder in a given health plan are placed out of home in restrictive placements (i.e., psychiatric hospital, residential treatment center, or incarcerated).

E. Outcomes/effectiveness framework

1. Maximization of treatment participation
2. Reduction or stabilization of symptoms
3. Improvement of level of functioning of child
4. Improvement of quality of life for child
5. Improvement of quality of life for family
6. Minimization of social and economic costs
7. Minimization of restrictive care

E.1.   Specific area: Maximization of treatment participation

E.1.1   **Recommendation/goal:** Efforts should be made to maximize treatment participation for children and families receiving treatment.

The importance of family involvement throughout all phases of assessment and treatment has been increasingly supported and valued as an important dimension in working with emotionally disturbed children and adolescents. To date, the evidence base that documents positive effects of family involvement and participation is limited. One study suggests the importance of family involvement in improving the school performance of chronically disruptive youths (130). Findings from another study support the benefits of parent involvement in early childhood programs (131). Ongoing work by Frieson, Korloff, and associates at the Portland State University Research and Training Center on Family Support and Children's Mental Health is attempting to demonstrate the effects of family participation and involvement on outcomes.

E.1.1.1   *Sample indicator:* Children and families participate in the decision to terminate treatment in a health plan.

Health plans always have some percentage of children and families who leave treatment before achieving reduction in symptoms or improvement in functioning. These treatment terminations are often referred to as "drop-outs." It is important for health plans to examine these terminations in an effort to understand whether the child and family were active participants with the treating clinician(s) in making the decision to terminate treatment.

E.1.1.1   **Sample measure:** Data will be collected about the number of children and families who participated in the decision to terminate treatment.

E.1.1.1   **Sample standard:** Estimate that 60% of records for patients who terminate treatment with the health plan contain documentation that the termination was planned and mutually agreed on by the child, family, and provider.

The numerator proposed for this measure is the number of records that contain documentation that there was planning and mutual agreement about the termination of treatment. The denominator is the total number of children and families who terminate treatment with the plan. Data would be collected from a random sample record review of patients who terminated treatment during the prior 12 months. It is recognized that review of individual records by a health plan is time intensive and may represent a practical limitation for this indicator. The suggested standard of 60% is based on clinical judgment and may need to be refined.

E.2. Specific area: Reduction and/or stabilization of symptoms

E.2.1   **Recommendation/goal:**   Children and adolescents receiving treatment known to be clinically effective for their condition(s) should experience a significant reduction in symptoms/signs after receiving appropriate treatment for a reasonable period of time.

E.2.1.1   *Sample indicator:* Reduction in symptoms of inattention, impulsivity, and hyperactivity among patients with the diagnosis of ADHD receiving treatment for the disorder in a given health plan.

Attention-deficit/hyperactivity disorder is a common psychiatric condition in children and adolescents. The diagnosis of ADHD requires a comprehensive assessment. Treatment for ADHD should be multimodal and targeted at reducing symptoms and improving overall functioning (72). Modalities for which there is evidence of efficacy and effectiveness in the treatment of ADHD include stimulant medications, parent training, behavior therapy, and combination multimodal treatment (61, 66–67). Comorbid psychiatric conditions may also have influences on treatment and must be considered in treatment planning and evaluation of outcomes.

E.2.1.1   **Sample measure:** Score on standardized ADHD rating scale.

E.2.1.1   **Sample standard:** Estimate 80% of patients receiving treatment will show a significant improvement in their score on a standardized rating scale within 4 months.

The numerator proposed for this measure is the number of children receiving treatment for ADHD who show significant improvement on the standardized rating scale. The denominator is the total number of children receiving treatment for ADHD in the plan. This indicator presumes that a standardized rating scale is used at the beginning of treatment and repeated at intervals during the course of treatment. Data would be collected from a random sample record review of patients with the DSM-IV-TR diagnosis of ADHD. It is recognized that review of individual records by a health plan is time intensive and may represent a practical limitation for this indicator. As an alternative to record reviews, health plans may use administrative data from their MIS if it includes data from rating scales. The suggested standard of 80% is based on clinical judgment and may need to be refined. A definition of "significant improvement" on the standardized rating scale would also need to be quantified.

An example of a standardized rating scale is the Clinical Global Impressions Scale (CGI) (132). The CGI has been used in ADHD medication studies to assess change. Examples of other scales useful in assessing change and improvement are the Connors Teacher Rating Scale—Revised (CTRS-R) and the Connors Parent Rating Scale—Revised (CPRS-R).

E.2.1.2   *Sample indicator:* Reduced use of substances among patients with a diagnosis of a substance-related disorder (abuse or dependence) who are receiving treatment for the disorder in a given health plan.

Substance use and abuse (i.e., alcohol and illegal drugs) remain a significant problem among children and adolescents. Reducing impairment related to substance abuse has been included as an outcome indicator in several leading measurement sets (MHSIP, AMBHA-PERMS, USDHHS-PPG). It was also identified as an important outcome indicator for children and adolescents by the American College of Mental Health Administration at the Santa Fe Summit on Behavioral Health (133–134). The primary goal of treatment is to achieve and maintain abstinence from the substance (74, 135). Comorbid psychiatric conditions (e.g., conduct disorder, oppositional defiant disorder) may have influences on treatment and must be considered in treatment planning and evaluation of outcomes.

E.2.1.2   **Sample measure:** Percentage of adolescent patients who started an intensive substance abuse treatment program who are abstaining from substance use (sober) in the sixth month of their aftercare program.

E.2.1.2   **Sample standard:** Estimate 40% of adolescent patients who started an intensive substance abuse treatment program will be abstaining from substance use (sober) in the sixth month of their aftercare program.

The numerator proposed for this measure is the number of adolescents who started an intensive substance abuse treatment program who are abstaining from substance use (sober) in the sixth month of their aftercare program. As a means to measure sobriety, patient reports, reports of family and other caregivers, and laboratory tests such as urinalysis may be considered. The denominator is the total number of adolescents who started an intensive substance abuse treatment program in the plan. Data would be collected from a random sample record review of patients with the DSM-IV-TR diagnosis of substance-related disorder who entered the intensive substance abuse treatment program in the prior 12 months. It is recognized that review of individual records by a health plan is time intensive and may represent a practical limitation for this indicator. The suggested standard of 40% is based on clinical judgment and may need to be refined.

E.3. Specific area: Improved level of functioning of the child

E.3.1   **Recommendation/goal:**   The level of functioning for children and adolescents receiving treatment known to be effective for their condition(s) should improve after receiving appropriate treatment for a reasonable period of time.

An important quality outcome indicator is level of functioning. Children and adolescents with psychiatric disorders frequently have impaired functioning in multiple life areas, including school, home and family, interpersonal relationships, and behavior in the community. Although available treatments can effectively reduce clinical symptoms for many children and adolescents, impairment in functioning may remain.

Improved level of functioning has been included as an outcome indicator in several leading measurement sets (MHSIP, AMBHA-PERMS, USDHHS-PPG). It was also identified as an important outcome indicator for children and adolescents by the American College of Mental Health Administration at the Santa Fe Summit on Behavioral Health (133–134).

E.3.1.1   *Sample indicator:* Improved school attendance for children and adolescents receiving treatment for a psychiatric disorder in a given health plan.

Improving attendance, behavioral functioning, and academic performance in school is specifically included as an outcome indicator in MHSIP. It was also identified as an important outcome indicator for children and adolescents by the American College of Mental Health Administration at the Santa Fe Summit on Behavioral Health (133–134).

This indicator is focused on those children and adolescents receiving mental health treatment in the plan who have a history of missing an average of 5 days or more per month of school.

E.3.1.1   **Sample measure:** For children with a history of missing school (as defined above), the number of days missed for any reason will be collected by the health plan from school records and caregiver reports.

E.3.1.1   **Sample standard:** Estimate 70% of patients with a history of missing school (as defined above) who are receiving mental health treatment in the plan will have a reduction in the number of missed days from school within 6 months.

The numerator proposed for this measure is the number of children with a history of missing school (as defined above) who are receiving mental health treatment in the plan and who have a reduction in the number of missed days from school for any reason. The denominator is the number of children with a history of missing school (as defined above) receiving treatment in the health plan. Data would be collected from a random sample of interviews with caregivers with a child or adolescent served by the plan during a 12-month period. This indicator presumes that baseline data on average number of days missed from school per month are collected at the beginning of treatment and subsequently at intervals (e.g., every 3–6 months) during the course of treatment. It is recognized that interviews of individual caregivers by a health plan are time intensive and may represent a practical limitation for this indicator. Alternatively, plans could develop a form to collect this information directly from the school. The suggested standard of 70% is based on clinical judgment and may need to be refined.

E.3.1.2   *Sample indicator:* Decreased involvement (i.e., arrests, detentions, or incarcerations) with juvenile justice/criminal system for children and adolescents receiving treatment for a psychiatric disorder in a health plan.

Involvement with the legal system has been included as an outcome indicator in several leading measurement sets (MHSIP, AMBHA-PERMS, USDHHS-PPG). It was also identified as an important outcome indicator for children and adolescents by the American College of Mental Health Administration at the Santa Fe Summit on Behavioral Health (133–134). It is expected that health plans will take appropriate steps and measures to minimize involvement with juvenile justice and criminal justice system for enrollees. This would include, but not be limited to, coordinating services with juvenile justice agencies, providing overall coordination of care, and providing necessary and appropriate support services to parents and families.

It is recognized that many factors are involved when children and adolescents become involved in the juvenile justice system. Often, the circumstances go beyond the influence that individual clinicians or health plans can have on the outcomes. Nevertheless, with these caveats, this indicator might be used as one measure of a plan's performance and also to make comparisons between health plans.

E.3.1.2   **Sample measure:** For children and adolescents with a history of documented involvement with the juvenile justice system, data about the number of arrests, severity of crimes, and number/length of incarcerations will be collected by the health plan from youth, caregivers, and juvenile justice authorities (local and state).

E.3.1.2   **Sample standard:** Number of documented arrests and incarcerations in a given time interval will be lower than the number in a comparable pretreatment interval.

Data on the number of arrests and incarcerations will be gathered for children and adolescents who are receiving treatment for a psychiatric disorder and have a history of documented arrests and incarcerations. Data would be collected from a random sample of caregivers with a child or adolescent served by the plan during a 12-month period. It is recognized that interviews of individual caregivers by a health plan are time intensive and may represent a practical limitation for this indicator.

E.3.1.3   *Sample indicator:* Children and adolescents diagnosed with a psychotic disorder receiving treatment for the disorder will demonstrate an improved level of functioning.

Psychotic disorders (e.g., schizophrenia) are not common in children and adolescents. The diagnosis of any psychotic disorder requires a comprehensive assessment conducted by a provider who specializes in diagnosing and treating children and adolescents. Treatment for any psychotic disorder should be multimodal and targeted at reducing symptoms and improving overall functioning (75, 136). Both antipsychotic and mood-stabilizing medications have been shown to be efficacious and effective in treating symptoms of psychotic disorders (61, 66).

E.3.1.3   **Sample measure:** Percentage of patients with a psychotic disorder diagnosis receiving treatment who show an improved level of functioning on a standardized functional assessment rating instrument within 6 months of treatment.

E.3.1.3   **Sample standard:** Estimate 80% of patients with a psychotic disorder diagnosis receiving treatment will show an improved level of functioning within 6 months of treatment.

The numerator proposed for this measure is the number of children receiving treatment for a psychotic disorder who show improvement on a standardized functional assessment instrument. The denominator is the total number of children receiving treatment for a psychotic disorder in the plan. This indicator presumes that a standardized functional assessment scale is used at the beginning of treatment and repeated at intervals (e.g., every 3 months) during the course of treatment. Examples of functional assessment scales include Child and Adolescent Functional Assessment Scale (98) and Child and Adolescent Needs and Strengths (137). Data would be collected from a random sample record review of patients with a DSM-IV diagnosis of one of the psychotic disorders who are treated during a 12-month period. It is recognized that review of individual records by a health plan is time intensive and may represent a practical limitation for this indicator. As an alternative to record reviews, health plans may use administrative data from their MIS if it includes data from rating scales. The suggested standard of 80% is based on clinical judgment and may need to be refined.

E.4.   Specific area: Improved quality of life for the child

E.4.1   **Recommendation/goal:** The quality of life for children and adolescents receiving treatment known to be effective for their condition(s) should improve after receiving appropriate treatment for a reasonable period of time.

Reporting positive changes resulting from treatment of a mental disorder has been included as an outcome indicator in several leading measurement sets (MHSIP, AMBHA-PERMS, USDHHS-PPG). Reporting a positive quality of life was specifically identified as an important outcome indicator for children and adolescents by the American College of Mental Health Administration at the Santa Fe Summit on Behavioral Health (133–134).

E.4.1.1   *Sample indicator:* Children and adolescents receiving treatment for a mental disorder report increased enjoyment of life and fuller participation in age- and/or developmentally appropriate activities.

E.4.1.1   **Sample measure:** The percentage of children and adolescents who report, through use of a standardized rating instrument, significant increase in their enjoyment of life.

E.4.1.1   **Sample standard:** Estimate 80% of children and adolescents receiving treatment in a given plan report significant increase in their enjoyment of life within 6 months of treatment.

The numerator proposed for this measure is the number of children receiving treatment for a mental disorder reported by caregivers to have a significant increase in their enjoyment of life on a valid quality-of-life assessment instrument. The denominator is the total number of children receiving treatment for a mental disorder in the plan. This indicator presumes that a standardized assessment instrument is used at the beginning of treatment and repeated at intervals during the course of treatment. An example of an instrument that can assess quality of life is the Child Health Questionnaire (CHQ) (138). The CHQ has three parent-completed versions and one child-completed version and can be used with children ages 5 and up. Data would be collected from a random sample record review of patients receiving treatment in the plan during a 12-month period. It is recognized that review of individual records by a health plan is time intensive and may represent a practical limitation for this indicator. As an alternative to record reviews, health plans may use administrative data from their MIS if it includes data from rating scales. The suggested standard of 80% is based on clinical judgment and may need to be refined.

E.4.2   **Recommendation/goal:** Children and adolescents undergoing treatment for mental illness have often experienced abuse and/or neglect prior to treatment in the health plan. Children and adolescents receiving treatment should be protected from criminal victimization, abuse, and/or neglect.

Being safe from criminal victimization, abuse, and neglect was specifically identified as an important outcome indicator for children and adolescents by the American College of Mental Health Administration at the Santa Fe Summit on Behavioral Health (133–134). It is expected that health plans will take appropriate steps and measures to minimize risk of abuse or neglect occurring with enrollees. This would include, but not be limited to, coordinating services with child protective service agencies, providing overall coordination of care, and providing necessary and appropriate support services to parents and families.

E.4.2.1   *Sample indicator:* Absence of documented abuse or neglect subsequent to the initiation of treatment of children in a given health plan.

It is recognized that many complex factors are involved when incidents of abuse or neglect occur with any child or adolescent. Most often, the circumstances go well beyond the influence that individual treating clinicians or health plans can have on these serious outcomes. It is also important to note that applying this specific indicator to a plan might lead to an unfair conclusion about a plan that serves a high proportion of the multiproblem patients and families with a higher incidence of abuse and neglect. In these situations, risk adjustment factors should be carefully considered. It is important to note also that all health care providers, teachers, child care workers, etc., are required by state law to report suspected child abuse/neglect (i.e., mandated reporters). However, keeping these caveats in mind, this indicator might be used as one measure of a plan's performance and also to make comparisons between health plans.

E.4.2.1   **Sample measure:** Data on the number of documented (founded) instances of abuse or neglect in a given time interval involving children receiving treatment will be collected by the health plan from child welfare/protective authorities (local and state).

E.4.2.1   **Sample standard:** Number of documented (founded) instances of abuse or neglect in a given time interval will be lower than the number in a comparable pretreatment interval.

Data on the number of documented (founded) instances of abuse or neglect will be gathered for children and adolescents who are receiving treatment and have a history of documented abuse or neglect. Data would be collected from a random sample record review of patients being treated with a history of documented abuse or neglect during a 12-month interval. It is recognized that review of individual records by a health plan is time intensive and may represent a practical limitation for this indicator. Alternatively, plans could develop a form to collect this information directly from the child welfare/protective authorities.

E.5.   Specific area: Improved quality of life for the child's family

E.5.1   **Recommendation/goal:** A family's quality of life should improve after their child has been receiving appropriate treatment of a mental disorder for a reasonable period of time.

Pediatric chronic physical illness and adult psychiatric disorders have been established as substantial sources of stress for family caregivers. To date, there is limited literature in the evidence base that addresses parental stress resulting from psychiatric disorders in children and adolescents. Lower quality of life has been reported by parents related to limited social support and other factors (139). Parents also experience more feelings of incompetence, depression, worries, and exhaustion, plus more problems with spouses and other family relationships (140).

E.5.1.1   *Sample indicator:* Reduction in family's stress level and impact of illness.

E.5.1.1   **Sample measure:** Percentage of families with children receiving treatment for a mental disorder who report a reduction in their stress level and impact of their child's illness using a standardized rating instrument.

E.5.1.1   **Sample standard:** Estimate 80% of families will show a reduction in their score on a standardized instrument within 6 months.

The numerator proposed for this measure is the number of families with children receiving treatment for a mental disorder who report reduction in their stress and burden level on a valid assessment instrument. The denominator is the total number of families with children receiving treatment for a mental disorder in the plan. This indicator presumes that a standardized assessment instrument is used at the beginning of treatment and repeated at intervals (e.g., every 3 or 6 months) during the course of treatment. Examples of instruments that can assess the family's stress level and impact of the child's illness are the Child and Adolescent Impact Assessment (CAIA) (141) and the Caregiver Strain Questionnaire (142).

Data would be collected from a random sample record review of patients receiving treatment in the plan during a 12-month period. It is recognized that review of individual records by a health plan is time intensive and may represent a practical limitation for this indicator. As an alternative to record reviews, health plans may use administrative data from their MIS if it includes data from rating scales. The suggested standard of 80% is based on clinical judgment and may need to be refined.

E.6.   Specific area: Minimization of social and economic costs

E.6.1   **Recommendation/goal:** Efforts should be made to minimize social and economic costs associated with psychiatric disorders in children and adolescents.

E.6.1.1   *Sample indicator:* Plans strive to limit the number of days of work missed by parents due to caring for a child receiving treatment for a mental disorder in a given health plan.

Pediatric chronic physical illness and adult psychiatric disorders have been established as substantial sources of burden for family caretakers. To date, there is limited literature in the evidence base which addresses the effects of psychiatric disorders in children and adolescents on their parents. Tracking days missed from work/employment has been included as an outcome indicator in several leading measurement sets (MHSIP, USDHHS-PPG). Parents' missing work to care for their child or adolescent with a mental disorder adds to the economic costs associated with the mental disorder.

E.6.1.1   **Sample measure:** Data about the number of parent days absent from work due to caring for a child receiving treatment will be collected by the health plan from caregiver reports.

E.6.1.1   **Sample standard:** Estimate less than 10% of parents with children receiving treatment in a health plan will have missed 20 or more days during a 12-month period.

The numerator proposed for this measure is the number of parents with children receiving treatment in health plan who are absent 20 or more days from work. The denominator is the total number of parents with children receiving treatment for a mental disorder in the plan. Data would be collected from a random sample of caregivers with a child or adolescent served by the plan during a 12-month period. It is recognized that interviews of individual caregivers by a health plan are time intensive and may represent a practical limitation for this indicator. Alternatively, plans could develop a form to collect this information from parents. The suggested standard of less than 10% being 20 or more days absent is based on clinical judgment and may need to be refined.

E.6.1.2   *Sample indicator:* Plans strive to limit the number of days of homebound instruction for children receiving treatment for a mental disorder in a given health plan.

Homebound instruction of a child or adolescent is not a substitute for their regular attendance and full participation in school. Children and adolescents with serious psychiatric disorders, however, are not infrequently removed from their regular school and provided with homebound instruction by the school system. Children receiving homebound instruction are separated from their classrooms and peers. Homebound instruction represents a less normative and more restrictive environment for the child. Improving attendance, functioning, and performance in school is specifically included as an outcome indicator in MHSIP. It was also identified as an important outcome indicator for children and adolescents by the American College of Mental Health Administration at the Santa Fe Summit on Behavioral Health (133–134). Reduction in homebound instruction should be associated with an increase in school attendance. It should also be noted, however, that homebound instruction may be necessary and preferable to no instruction when the child has been suspended or expelled from school.

E.6.1.2   **Sample measure:** The number of days of homebound instruction for children receiving treatment for a mental disorder will be collected from school and caregiver reports.

E.6.1.2   **Sample standard:** Estimate less than 10% of children receiving treatment for a mental disorder receive 30 or more days of homebound instruction during a 12-month period.

The numerator proposed for this measure is the number of children receiving treatment in health plans who have 30 or more days of homebound instruction. The denominator is the total number of children receiving treatment for a mental disorder in the plan. Data would be collected from a random sample of caregivers with a child or adolescent served by the plan. It is recognized that interviews of individual caregivers by a health plan are time intensive and may represent a practical limitation for this indicator. Alternatively, plans could develop a form to collect this information from parents and/or schools. The suggested standard of less than 10% is based on clinical judgment and may need to be refined.

E.7.   Specific area: Minimization of restrictive care

E.7.1   **Recommendation/goal:** Children and adolescents with mental illness should receive care and treatment in the least restrictive/most normative settings that are appropriate to their clinical needs.

The current evidence base demonstrates neither efficacy nor effectiveness for inpatient hospital treatment, and the limited evidence on residential treatment is weak and questionable (66). Out-of-home placement has been included as an outcome indicator in several leading measurement sets (MHSIP, USDHHS-PPG). Having a stable living situation in a home with a family was identified as an important outcome indicator for children and adolescents by the American College of Mental Health Administration at the Santa Fe Summit on Behavioral Health (133–134). It should be noted, however, that there are situations when out-of-home care is necessary. The intent of this recommendation and indicator is not to unnecessarily limit clinically necessary and appropriate out-of-home care, but rather to emphasize that health plans and families should work closely together and carefully consider any out-of-home treatment or placement decisions.

E.7.1.1   *Sample indicator:* Plans strive to limit the number of days children receiving treatment for a mental disorder in a given health plan are placed out-of-home in restrictive placements (i.e., psychiatric hospital, residential treatment center, or incarcerated).

E.7.1.1   **Sample measure:** Data about the number of days children receiving treatment are placed out-of-home in restrictive placements will be collected by the health plan from provider and caregiver reports.

E.7.1.1   **Sample standard:** Estimate less than 20% of children receiving treatment are placed out-of-home for 30 or more days in restrictive placements during a 12-month period.

The numerator proposed for this measure is the number of children receiving treatment for a mental disorder who are placed out-of-home for 30 or more days in restrictive placements. The denominator is the total number of children receiving treatment for a mental disorder in the plan. Data would be collected from a random sample of caregivers with a child or adolescent served by the plan during a 12-month period. The level of restrictiveness of placements can be rated using the Restrictiveness of Living Environment Scale (143). It is recognized that interviews of individual caregivers by a health plan are time intensive and may represent a practical limitation for this indicator. As an alternative to record reviews, health plans may use administrative data from their MIS if it includes data from rating scales. The suggested standard of less than 20% is based on clinical judgment and may need to be refined.

VI. Next Steps

The future use of the task force report will be the responsibility of the APA's Office of Quality Improvement and Psychiatric Services and the APA's Council on Quality Improvement.

The overall mission of the APA's Office of Quality Improvement and Psychiatric Services is to facilitate the optimal provision of quality psychiatric services, including substance abuse services. The office works

1) to document the scientific basis of psychiatric care through the development of practice guidelines, and 2) to advocate for strong standards for quality care through accreditation and related processes. Two important goals of the office are:

- To promote the use of scientifically valid data and accumulated clinical experience to inform the processes of clinical and policy decision making.
- To provide psychiatric leadership in the improvement of treatment by developing, commenting on, and disseminating quality improvement measures for use by clinicians, organized systems of care, accrediting bodies, and others.

The APA's Council on Quality Improvement includes the Steering Committee on Practice Guidelines; Committee on Standards and Survey Procedures; Committee on Quality Indicators; and Task Force on Quality Indicators for Children; and the Task Force on Patient Safety.

Promotion and Implementation of Indicators

A critical component of all of the APA's efforts related to quality improvement is the ongoing development of indicators, or measures, that accurately and appropriately reflect important aspects of the quality of care provided to children, adolescents, and their families.

Under the auspices of the APA's Council on Quality Improvement, the Committee on Quality Indicators will assume responsibility for the promotion and use of this report. Specifically, it is anticipated that the committee will

- Develop strategies to disseminate the indicators.
- Encourage additional research and field testing of indicators.
- Promote adoption of selected quality indicators by quality oversight organizations that are implementing measurement programs.

References

1. Hermann RC, Leff HS, Palmer RH, Yang D, Teller T, Provost S, Jakubiak C, Chan J: Quality measures for mental health care: results from a national inventory. Med Care Res Rev 2000; 57 (suppl 2):136-154

2. Institute of Medicine: Crossing the Quality Chasm: A New Health System for the 21st Century. Washington, DC, National Academy Press, 2001

3. Green M: Bright Futures: Guidelines for Health Supervision of Infants, Children, and Adolescents. Arlington, VA, National Center for Education in Maternal and Child Health, 1994

4. Health Care Financing Administration: State Medicaid Manual (HCFA Publ No 45). Washington, DC, Health Care Financing Administration, Part 5, Section 5123

5. Jellinek MS, Murphy JM: Use of pediatric symptom checklist to screen for psychosocial problems in pediatric primary care: a national feasibility study. Arch Pediatr Adolesc Med 153(3):254–260, 1999

6. Glascoe FP: Using parents' concerns to detect and address developmental and behavioral problems. J Soc Pediatr Nurs 4(1):24–35, 1999

7. Glascoe FP: Evidence-based approach to developmental and behavioral surveillance using parents' concerns. Child Care Health Dev 26(2):137–149, 2000

8. Johnson J, Harris E, Spitzer R, Williams J: The Patient Health Questionnaire for Adolescents: validation of an instrument for the assessment of mental disorders among primary care patients. Journal of Adolescent Health (in press)

9. Bird HR, Shaffer D, Fisher P, Gould MS, Staghezza B, Chen JY, Hoven C: The Columbia Impairment Scale (CIS): pilot findings on a measure of global impairment for children and adolescents. International Journal of Methods in Psychiatric Research 3:167–176, 1993

10. Lachar D, Klein R, Boersma D: Personality Inventory for Children: approaches to actuarial interpretation in clinic and school settings, in The Assessment of Child and Adolescent Personality. Edited by Knoff H. New York, Guilford, 1986, pp 273–308

11. Achenbach TM: Manual for the Child Behavior Checklist/4-18 and 1991 Profile. Burlington, University of Vermont, 1991

12. Achenbach TM: Manual for the Child Behavior Checklist/2-3 and 1992 Profile. Burlington, University of Vermont, 1992

13. Conners CK: Conners' Rating Scales—Revised: Technical Manual. New York, Multi-Health Systems, 1997

14. Kelsoe J: Mood disorders—genetics, in Kaplan and Sadock's Comprehensive Textbook of Psychiatry, 7th Edition. Edited by Sadock BJ, Sadock VA. Philadelphia, PA, Williams & Wilkins, 2000, pp 1308–1318

15. Field T: Infants of depressed mothers. Infant Behavior and Development 18:1–13, 1995

16. Field T, Grizzle N, Scafidi F, Abrams S, Richardson S: Massage therapy for infants of depressed mothers. Infant Behavior and Development 19:107–112, 1996

17. Beardslee W, Wright E, Rothberg PC, Salt P, Versage E: Response of families to two preventive intervention strategies: long-term differences in behavior and attitude change. J Am Acad Child Adolesc Psychiatry 35(6): 774–782, 1996

18. Beardslee W, Salt P, Versage E, Gladstone T, Wright E, Rothberg P: Sustained change in parents receiving preventive interventions for families with depression. Am J Psychiatry 154:510–515, 1997

19. Olds DL, Henderson CR Jr, Phelps C, Kitzman H, Hanks C: Effect of prenatal and infancy nurse home visitation on government spending. Med Care 31(2):155–174, 1993

20. Olds DL, Eckenrode J, Henderson CR Jr, Kitzman H, Powers J, Cole R, Sidora K, Morris P, Pettitt LM, Luckey D: Long-term effects of home visitation on maternal life course and child abuse and neglect. Fifteen-year follow-up of a randomized trial. JAMA 278(8):637–643, 1997

21. Field TM, Scafidi F, Pickens J, Prodromidis M, Pelaez-Nogueras M, Torquati J, Wilcox H, Malphurs J, Schanberg S, Kuhn C: Polydrug-using adolescent mothers and their infants receiving early intervention. Adolescence 33(129):117–143, 1998

22. Abdin RR. Parenting Stress Index, 3rd Edition: Professional Manual. Odessa, FL, Psychological Assessment Resources, 1995

23. Steiner H: Chronic illness and physical disabilities, in Handbook of Child and Adolescent Psychiatry, Vol 4. Edited by Noshpitz J, Alessi N. New York, Wiley, 1997, pp 251–273

24. Pearson DA, Pumariega AJ, Seilheimer DK: The development of psychiatric symptomatology in patients with cystic fibrosis. J Am Acad Child Adolesc Psychiatry 30(2):290–297, 1991

25. Pumariega A, Pearson D, Seilheimer D: Family and individual adjustment in children with cystic fibrosis. Journal of Child and Family Studies 2(2):109–118, 1993

26. Hummel L, Feinstein C: Developmental language disorders in school-age children, in Handbook of Child and Adolescent Psychiatry, Vol 2. Edited by Noshpitz J, Kernberg P, Bemporad J. New York, Wiley, 1997, pp 420–435

27. Pumariega AJ, Johnson NP, Sheridan D: Emotional disturbance and substance abuse in youth placed in residential group homes. Journal of Mental Health Administration 22(4):426–432, 1995

28. Atkins D, Pumariega A, Montgomery L, Rogers K, Nybro C, Jeffers G, Sease F: Mental health and incarcerated youth, I: prevalence and nature of psychopathology. Journal of Child and Family Studies 8(2):193–204, 1999

29. Otto R, Greenstein J, Johnson M, Friedman R: Prevalence of mental disorders among youth in the juvenile justice system: responding to the mental health needs of youth in the juvenile justice system. Seattle, WA, National Coalition for the Mentally Ill in the Criminal Justice System, 1992

30. Finney J, Riley A, Cataldo M: Psychology in primary care: effects of brief targeted therapy on children's medical care utilization. J Pediatr Psychol 16:447–461, 1991

31. Roter D, Hall J, Merisca R, Nordstrom B, Cretin D, Svardstad B: Effectiveness of interventions to improve patient compliance. Med Care 36:1138–1161, 1998

32. Pless IB, Feeley N, Gottlieb L, Rowat K, Dougherty G, Willard B: A randomized trial of a nursing intervention to promote the adjustment of children with chronic physical disorders. Pediatrics 94(1):70–75, 1994

33. Henggeler S, Mihalic S, Rone L, Thomas C, Timmons-Mitchell J: Multisystemic Therapy, 6th Edition. Boulder, CO, Center for the Study and Prevention of Violence, Institute of Behavioral Science, University of Colorado, 1998

34. Strayhorn J, Weidman C: Follow-up of one year after parent-child interaction training: effects of behavior of preschool children. J Am Acad Child Adolesc Psychiatry 30:138–143, 1991

35. Kellam SG, Rebok GW, Ialongo N, Mayer LS: The course and malleability of aggressive behavior from early first grade into middle school: results of a developmental epidemiologically-based preventive trial. J Child Psychol Psychiatry 35(2):259–281, 1994

36. U.S. Department of Health and Human Services: Youth Violence: A Report of the Surgeon General. Rockville, MD, National Center for Injury Prevention and Control, Centers for Disease Control and Prevention; Center for Mental Health Services, Substance Abuse and Mental Health Services Administration; and National Institute of Mental Health, National Institutes of Health, 2001

37. Grisso T, Barnum R, Fletcher K, Cauffman E, Peuschold D: Massachusetts youth screening instrument for mental health needs of juvenile justice youths. J Am Acad Child Adolesc Psychiatry 40(5):541–548, 2001

38. Grisso T, Barnum R: Massachusetts Youth Screening Instrument: Users Manual and Technical Report, 2nd Version. Worcester, University of Massachusetts Medical School, 2000

39. Greenberg T, Domitrovich C, Bumbarger B: Preventing mental disorders in school-age children: a review of the effectiveness of prevention programs. Rockville, MD, Center for Mental Health Services, Substance Abuse and Mental Health Administration, 1999

40. Spence S, Dadds M: Preventing childhood anxiety disorders. Journal of Behavior Change 13:241–249, 1996

41. Hains A, Ellman S: Stress inoculation training as a preventive intervention for high school youth. Journal of Cognitive Psychotherapy 8:219–232, 1994

42. Klingman A, Hochdorf Z: Coping with distress and self harm: the impact of a primary prevention program among adolescents 2. J Adolesc 16(2): 121–140, 1993

43. Orbach I, Bar-Joseph H: The impact of a suicide prevention program for adolescents on suicidal tendencies, hopelessness, ego identity, and coping. Suicide Life Threat Behav 23(2):120–129, 1993

44. Ollendick TH, Weist MD, Borden MC, Greene RW: Sociometric status and academic, behavioral, and psychological adjustment: a five-year longitudinal study. J Consult Clin Psychol 60:80–87, 1992

45. Lochman J, Coie J, Underwood M, Terry R: Effectiveness of a social relations intervention program for aggressive and nonaggressive, rejected children. J Consult Clin Psychol 61(6):1053–1058, 1993

46. Hudley C, Graham S: School-based interventions for aggressive African-American boys. Applied and Preventive Psychology 4:185–195, 1995

47. Killen JD, Taylor CB, Hammer LD, Litt I, Wilson DM, Rich T, Hayward C, Simmonds B, Kraemer H, Varady A: An attempt to modify unhealthful eating attitudes and weight regulation practices of young adolescent girls. Int J Eat Disord 13(4):369–384, 1993

48. Levine M, Hill L: A Five Day Lesson Plan on Eating Disorders: Grades 7–12. Columbus, OH, National Eating Disorders Organization, 1991

49. Moriarty D, Shore R, Maxim N: Evaluation of an eating disorders curriculum. Eval Program Plann 13:407–413, 1990

50. Shisslak C, Crago M, Neal M: Prevention of eating disorders among adolescents. American Journal of Health Promotion 5:100–106, 1990

51. Clarke GN, Hawkins W, Murphy M, Sheeber LB, Lewinsohn PM, Seeley JR: Targeted prevention of unipolar depressive disorder in an at-risk sample of high school adolescents: a randomized trial of a group cognitive intervention. J Am Acad Child Adolesc Psychiatry 34(3):312–321, 1995

52. Tremblay RE, Pagani-Kurtz L, Masse LC, Vitaro F, Pihl RO: A bimodal preventive intervention for disruptive kindergarten boys: its impact through mid-adolescence. J Consult Clin Psychol 63(4):560–568, 1995

53. Olds DL, Henderson CR Jr, Cole R, Eckenrode J, Kitzman H, Luckey D, Pettitt L, Sidora K, Morris P, Powers J: Long-term effects of nurse home visitation on children's criminal and antisocial behavior: 15-year follow-up of a randomized controlled trial. JAMA 280(14):1238–1244, 1998

54. Webster-Stratton C: The Incredible Years Training Series (Juvenile Justice Bulletin). Washington, DC, Office of Juvenile Justice and Delinquency Prevention, Office of Justice Programs, U.S. Department of Justice, 2000

55. Elliott DS: Blueprints for violence prevention. http://www.colorado.edu/cspv/blueprints/contacts.htm. Boulder, Center for the Study and Prevention of Violence (CSPV), Institute of Behavioral Science, University of Colorado, 1998

56. Elliott D, Hamburg BA, Williams KR: Violence in American Schools: A New Perspective. Cambridge, UK, Cambridge University Press, 1998

57. American Academy of Child and Adolescent Psychiatry: Practice parameters for the assessment and treatment of children and adolescents with depressive disorders. J Am Acad Child Adolesc Psychiatry 37(10, suppl): 63S–83S, 1998

58. American Academy of Child and Adolescent Psychiatry: Practice parameters for the psychiatric assessment of children and adolescents. J Am Acad Child Adolesc Psychiatry 36 (10, suppl):4S–20S, 1997

59. American Academy of Child and Adolescent Psychiatry: Practice parameters for the psychiatric assessment of infants and toddlers (0–36 months). J Am Acad Child Adolesc Psychiatry 36 (10, suppl):21S–36S, 1997

60. New York State Office of Mental Health: Children's Special Needs Plans Request for Information. Albany, Division of Managed Care, Bureau of Performance and Outcomes Management, New York State Office of Mental Health, 1998

61. Weisz JR, Jenson PR: Efficacy and effectiveness of child and adolescent psychotherapy and pharmacotherapy. Mental Health Services Research 1(3):125–157, 1999

62. Brestan EV, Eyberg SM: Effective psychosocial treatments of conduct-disordered children and adolescents: 29 years, 82 studies, and 5,272 kids. J Clin Child Psychol 27(2):180–189, 1998

63. Kaslow NJ, Thompson MP: Applying the criteria for empirically supported treatments to studies of psychosocial interventions for child and adolescent depression. J Clin Child Psychol 27(2):146–155, 1998

64. Pelham WE Jr, Wheeler T, Chronis A: Empirically supported psychosocial treatments for attention deficit hyperactivity disorder. Clin Child Psychol 27(2):190–205, 1998

65. Ollendick TH, King NJ: Empirically supported treatments for children with phobic and anxiety disorders: current status. J Clin Child Psychol 27(2):156–167, 1998

66. Burns B, Hoagwood K, Mrazek P: Effective treatment for mental disorders in children and adolescents. Clinical Child and Family Psychology Review 2(4):199–254, 1999

67. Burns BJ, Compton SN, Egger HL, Farmer EMZ: An annotated review of the evidence base for psychosocial and psychopharmacological interventions for children with attention-deficit/hyperactivity disorder, major depressive disorder, disruptive behavior disorders, anxiety disorders, and post traumatic stress disorder: Durham, NC, Duke University Medical Center, 2000

68. American Academy of Child and Adolescent Psychiatry: Practice parameters for the assessment and treatment of children and adolescents with bipolar disorder. J Am Acad Child Adolesc Psychiatry 36 (10, suppl): 157S–158S, 1997

69. American Academy of Child and Adolescent Psychiatry: Practice parameters for the assessment and treatment of children and adolescents with obsessive-compulsive disorder. J Am Acad Child Adolesc Psychiatry 37 (10, suppl):27S–45S, 1998

70. American Academy of Child and Adolescent Psychiatry: Practice parameters for the assessment and treatment of children and adolescents with posttraumatic stress disorder. J Am Acad Child Adolesc Psychiatry 37 (10, suppl):4S–26S, 1998

71. American Academy of Child and Adolescent Psychiatry: Practice parameters for the assessment and treatment of children and adolescents with anxiety disorders. J Am Acad Child Adolesc Psychiatry 36 (10, suppl): 69S–84S, 1997

72. American Academy of Child and Adolescent Psychiatry: Practice parameters for the assessment and treatment of children, adolescents, and adults with attention-deficit/hyperactivity disorder. J Am Acad Child Adolesc Psychiatry 36 (10, suppl):85S–121S, 1997

73. American Academy of Child and Adolescent Psychiatry: Practice parameters for the assessment and treatment of children and adolescents with conduct disorder. J Am Acad Child Adolesc Psychiatry 36 (10, suppl): 122S–139S, 1997

74. American Academy of Child and Adolescent Psychiatry: Practice parameters for the assessment and treatment of children and adolescents with substance use disorders. J Am Acad Child Adolesc Psychiatry 36 (10, suppl):140S–156S, 1997

75. American Academy of Child and Adolescent Psychiatry: Practice parameters for the assessment and treatment of children and adolescents with schizophrenia. J Am Acad Child Adolesc Psychiatry 36 (10, suppl):177S–193S, 1997

76. Jobson KO, Potter WZ: International Psychopharmacology Algorithm Project report. Psychopharmacol Bull 31(3):457–459, 1995

77. Klein RG: The role of methylphenidate in psychiatry. Arch Gen Psychiatry 52(6):429–433, 1995

78. Jacobvitz D, Sroufe LA, Stewart M, Leffert N: Treatment of attentional and hyperactivity problems in children with sympathomimetic drugs: a comprehensive review. J Am Acad Child Adolesc Psychiatry 29(5):677–688, 1990

79. Swanson JM: Effect of stimulant medication on children with attention deficit disorder: a "review of reviews." Special Issue: Issues in the Education of Children With Attentional Deficit Disorder. Exceptional Children 60(2):154–161, 1993

80. MTA Cooperative Group: Moderators and mediators of treatment response for children with attention-deficit/hyperactivity disorder: the Multimodal Treatment Study of Children With Attention-Deficit/Hyperactivity Disorder. Arch Gen Psychiatry 56(12):1088–1096, 1999

81. MTA Cooperative Group: A 14-month randomized clinical trial of treatment strategies for attention-deficit/hyperactivity disorder: Multimodal Treatment Study of Children With ADHD. Arch Gen Psychiatry 56(12): 1073–1086, 1999

82. Leonard HL, Swedo SE, Rapoport JL, Koby EV, Lenane MC, Cheslow DL, Hamburger SD: Treatment of obsessive-compulsive disorder with clomipramine and desipramine in children and adolescents: a double-blind crossover comparison. Arch Gen Psychiatry 46(12):1088–1092, 1989

83. Flament MF, Rapoport JL, Berg CJ, Sceery W, Kilts C, Mellstrom B, Linnoila M: Clomipramine treatment of childhood obsessive-compulsive disorder: a double-blind controlled study. Arch Gen Psychiatry 42(10): 977–983, 1985

84. DeVeaugh-Geiss J, Moroz G, Biederman J, Cantwell D, Fontaine R, Greist JH, Reichler R, Katz R, Landau P: Clomipramine hydrochloride in childhood and adolescent obsessive-compulsive disorder: a multicenter trial. J Am Acad Child Adolesc Psychiatry 31(1):45–49, 1992

85. Riddle MA, Scahill L, King RA, Hardin MT, Anderson GM, Ort SI, Smith JC, Leckman JF, Cohen DJ: Double-blind, crossover trial of fluoxetine and placebo in children and adolescents with obsessive-compulsive disorder. J Am Acad Child Adolesc Psychiatry 31(6):1062–1069, 1992

86. March JS, Kobak KA, Jefferson JW, Mazza J, Greist JH: A double-blind, placebo-controlled trial of fluvoxamine versus imipramine in outpatients with major depression. J Clin Psychiatry 51(5):200–202, 1990

87. March JS, Biederman J, Wolkow R, Safferman A, Mardekian J, Cook EH, Cutler NR, Dominguez R, Ferguson J, Muller B, Riesenberg R, Rosenthal M, Sallee FR, Wagner KD, Steiner H: Sertraline in children and adolescents with obsessive-compulsive disorder: a multicenter randomized controlled trial. JAMA 280(20):1752–1756, 1998

88. Emslie GJ, Rush AJ, Weinberg WA, Kowatch RA, Hughes CW, Carmody T, Rintelmann J: A double-blind, randomized, placebo-controlled trial of fluoxetine in children and adolescents with depression. Arch Gen Psychiatry 54(11):1031–1037, 1997

89. American Academy of Child and Adolescent Psychiatry: Practice parameters for the assessment and treatment of children, adolescents, and adults with autism and other pervasive developmental disorders. J Am Acad Child Adolesc Psychiatry 38 (10, suppl):32S–54S, 1999

90. American Academy of Child and Adolescent Psychiatry: Practice parameters for the assessment and treatment of children, adolescents, and adults with mental retardation and comorbid mental disorders. J Am Acad Child Adolesc Psychiatry 38 (10, suppl):5S–31S, 1999

91. American Academy of Child and Adolescent Psychiatry: Practice parameters for the assessment and treatment of children and adolescents with language and learning disorders. J Am Acad Child Adolesc Psychiatry 37 (10, suppl):46S–62S, 1998

92. U.S. Department of Health and Human Services. Mental Health: A Report of the Surgeon General. Rockville, MD, Center for Mental Health Services, Substance Abuse and Mental Health Services Administration; National Institute of Mental Health, National Institutes of Health, 1999

93. American Academy of Child and Adolescent Psychiatry: Best Principles for Managed Care Medicaid RFP's: How Decision-Makers Can Select and Monitor High Quality Programs! Washington, DC, American Academy of Child and Adolescent Psychiatry, 1998

94. American Academy of Child and Adolescent Psychiatry: Best Principles for Managing Outcomes in Managed Medicaid Programs. Washington, DC, American Academy of Child and Adolescent Psychiatry, 1999

95. Smith LS: Concept analysis: cultural competence. J Cult Divers 5(1):4–10, 1998

96. Kleinman A: Anthropology and psychiatry: the role of culture in cross-cultural research on illness. Br J Psychiatry 151:447–454, 1987

97. Schlenger WE, Etheridge RM, Hansen DJ, Fairbank DW, Onken J: Evaluation of state efforts to improve systems of care for children and adolescents with severe emotional disturbances: The CASSP (Child and Adolescent Service System Program) Initial Cohort Study. Journal of Mental Health Administration 19(2):131–142, 1992

98. Rush JA Jr, Pincus HA, First MB, Blacker D, Endicott J, Keith SJ, Phillips KA, Ryan ND, Smith GR Jr, Tsuang MT, Widiger TA, Zarin DA: Handbook of Psychiatric Measures. Washington, DC, American Psychiatric Association, 2000, pp 278–361

99. Mufson L, Weissman MM, Moreau D, Garfinkel R: Efficacy of interpersonal psychotherapy for depressed adolescents. Arch Gen Psychiatry 56(6):573–579, 1999

100. Starfield B: Primary Care. New York, Oxford University Press, 1998, p 145
101. National Committee on Quality Assurance: Standards for the accreditation of MCO's, effective July 1, 2000 –June 30, 2001. Washington, DC, National Committee on Quality Assurance, 1999
102. Carr-Hill RA: The measurement of patient satisfaction. J Public Health Med 14(3):236–249, 1992
103. Hall JA, Dornan MC: Meta-analysis of satisfaction with medical care: description of research domain and analysis of overall satisfaction levels. Soc Sci Med 27(6):637–644, 1988
104. Marshall GN, Wells KB, Sherbourne CD, Hays RD: The structure of patient satisfaction with outpatient medical care. Psychological Assessment 5:477–483, 1993
105. Strasser S, Aharony L, Greenberger D: The patient satisfaction process: moving toward a comprehensive model. Med Care Rev 50(2):219–248, 1993
106. Litt IF: Satisfaction with health care: the adolescent's perspective (editorial). J Adolesc Health 23(2):59–60, 1998
107. Kuhlthau K, Walker DK, Perrin JM, Bauman L, Gortmaker SL, Newacheck PW, Stein RE: Assessing managed care for children with chronic conditions. Health Aff (Millwood) 17(4):42–52, 1998
108. Hennelly VD, Boxerman SB: Out-of-plan use and disenrollment: outgrowths of dissatisfaction with a prepaid group plan. Med Care 21(3):348–359, 1983
109. Davies AR, Ware JE Jr, Brook RH, Peterson JR, Newhouse JP: Consumer acceptance of prepaid and fee-for-service medical care: results from a randomized controlled trial. Health Serv Res 21(3):429–452, 1986
110. Aharony L, Strasser S: Patient satisfaction: what we know about and what we still need to explore. Med Care Rev 50(1):49–79, 1993
111. Rubin HR, Gandek B, Rogers WH, Kosinski M, McHorney CA, Ware JE Jr: Patients' ratings of outpatient visits in different practice settings: results from the Medical Outcomes Study. JAMA 270(7):835–840, 1993
112. Greenley JR, Robitschek CG: Evaluation of a comprehensive program for youth with severe emotional disorders: an analysis of family experiences and satisfaction. Am J Orthopsychiatry 61(2):291–297, 1991
113. Loff CD, Trigg LJ, Cassels C: An evaluation of consumer satisfaction in a child psychiatric service: viewpoints of patients and parents. Am J Orthopsychiatry 57(1):132–134, 1987
114. Byalin K: Assessing parental satisfaction with children's mental health services: a pilot study. Evaluation and Program Planning 16:69–72, 1993
115. Heflinger CA, Sonnichsen SE, Brannan AM: Parent satisfaction with children's mental health services in a children's mental health managed care demonstration. Journal of Mental Health Administration 23(1):69–79, 1996

116. Brannan A, Sonnichsen SE, Heflinger C: Reliability and validity of scales to measure parent satisfaction with children's mental health services. AHSR & FHSR Annual Meeting Abstract Book 12:75–76, 1995

117. Shapiro JP, Welker CJ, Jacobson BJ: The Youth Client Satisfaction Questionnaire: development, construct validation, and factor structure. J Clin Child Psychol 26(1):87–98, 1997

118. Schwab ME, Stone K: Conceptual and methodologic issues in the evaluation of children's satisfaction with their mental health care. Evaluation and Program Planning 6(3–4):283–289, 1983

119. Young SC, Nicholson J, Davis M: An overview of issues in research on consumer satisfaction with child and adolescent mental health services. Journal of Child and Family Studies 4:219–238, 1995

120. Garland AF, Besinger BA: Adolescents' perceptions of outpatient mental health services. Journal of Child and Family Studies 5:355–375, 1996

121. Freed LH, Ellen JM, Irwin CE Jr, Millstein SG: Determinants of adolescents' satisfaction with health care providers and intentions to keep follow-up appointments. J Adolesc Health 22(6):475–479, 1998

122. Jerrell JM: Utilization management analysis for children's mental health services. J Behav Health Serv Res 25(1):35–42, 1998

123. Eisen SV, Shaul JA, Clarridge B, Nelson D, Spink J, Cleary PD: Development of a consumer survey for behavioral health services. Psychiatr Serv 50(6):793–798, 1999

124. Shaul JA, Eisen SV, Stringfellow VL, Clarridge BR, Hermann RC, Nelson D, Anderson E, Kubrin AI, Leff HS, Cleary PD: Use of consumer ratings for quality improvement in behavioral health insurance plans. Joint Commission Journal of Quality Improvement 27(4):216–229, 2001

125. Switzer G, Scholle S, Johnson B, Kelleher K: The client cultural competence inventory: an instrument for assessing cultural competence in behavioral managed care organizations. Journal of Child and Family Studies 7(4):483–491, 1998

126. Tirado MD: Tools for Monitoring Cultural Competence: Final Report to the Office of Planning and Evaluation, Health Resources and Services Administration, 1996

127. LaFromboise T, Coleman H, Hernandez A: Development and factor structure of the Cross-Cultural Counseling Inventory—Revised. Professional Psychology: Research and Practice 22(5):380–388, 1991

128. Stuntzer-Gibson D, Koren PE, DeChillo N: The Youth Satisfaction Questionnaire (YSQ): what kids think of services. Families in Society 76:616–624, 1995

129. Lee M. Parent Assessment of Care Survey (PACS). Albany, Bureau of Performance and Outcomes Management. New York State Office of Mental Health, 2000

130. Aeby V, Manning B, Thyer B, Carpenter-Aeby T: Comparing outcomes of an alternative school program offered with and without intensive family involvement. The School Community Journal 9(1):17–31, 1999

131. Miedel WT, Reynolds AJ: Parent involvement in early intervention for disadvantaged children: does it matter? Journal of School Psychology 37(4):379–402, 1999

132. Guy W: ECDEU Assessment Manual for Psychopharmacology— Revised (DHEW Publ No ADM 76-338, 218-222). Rockville, MD, U.S. Department of Health, Education, and Welfare, Public Health Service, Alcohol, Drug Abuse, and Mental Health Administration, NIMH Psychopharmacology Research Branch, Division of Extramural Research Programs, 1976

133. American College of Mental Health Administration: A comparative analysis of behavioral health performance/outcome indicator set, in Santa Fe Summit on Behavioral Health—Preserving Quality and Value in the Managed Care Equation, 1997, Appendix 5, pp 107–132

134. American College of Mental Health Administration: Outcomes measurement for children and adolescents with SED, in Santa Fe Summit on Behavioral Health—Preserving Quality and Value in the Managed Care Equation, 1997, Section 3, pp 21–26

135. American Psychiatric Association: Practice guideline for treatment of patients with substance use disorders: alcohol, cocaine, opioids. Am J Psychiatry 152 (11, suppl):1–59, 1995

136. American Psychiatric Association: Practice guideline for the treatment of patients with schizophrenia. Am J Psychiatry 154(4):1–63, 1997

137. Lyons JS, Sokol PT, Khalsa A, Lee M: Child and Adolescent Needs and Strengths for Children With Mental Health Challenges (CANS-MH) Manual. Winnetka, IL, Buddin Praed Foundation, 1999

138. Landgraf JM, Abetz L, Ware JE: The CHQ's User Manual. Boston, MA, Health Institute, New England Medical Center, 1996

139. Crowley MJ, Kazdin AE: Child psychosocial functioning and parent quality of life among clinically referred children. Journal of Child and Family Studies 7: 233–251, 1998

140. Farmer EMZ, Burns BJ, Angold A, Costello EJ: Impact of children's mental health problems on families: relationships with service use. Journal of Emotional and Behavioral Disorders 5(4):230–238. 1997

141. Angold A, Patrick KS, Burns BJ, Costello E: The Child and Adolescent Impact Assessment (CAIA), Version 2.0. Durham, NC, Department of Psychiatry and Behavioral Sciences, Duke University, 1999

142. Brannan A, Heflinger C, Bickman L: The Caregiver Strain Questionnaire: measuring the impact on the family of living with a child with serious emotional disturbance. Journal of Emotional and Behavioral Disorders 5(4):212–222, 1997

143. Hawkins RP, Alameida MC, Fabry B, Reitz AL: A scale to measure restrictiveness of living environment for troubled children and youth. Hosp Community Psychiatry 43:54–58, 1992

Acronyms and Abbreviations

AACAP American Academy of Child and Adolescent Psychiatry
AAHCC American Accreditation Healthcare Commission
ACMHA American College of Mental Health Administration
AHCPR Agency for Health Care Policy and Research (renamed Agency for Healthcare Research and Quality)
AMAP American Medical Accreditation Program (no longer exists)
AMBHA American Managed Behavioral Health Association
APA American Psychiatric Association

BHMAP Behavioral Health Measurement Advisory Panel

CAHPS Consumer Assessment for Health Plans Study
CASSP Child and Adolescent Service System Program
CBCL Child Behavior Checklist
CBT Cognitive-behavioral therapy
CMHS Center for Mental Health Services
CMS Centers for Medicare and Medicaid Services (formerly HCFA)
CQI Continuous Quality Improvement
CSNP Children's Special Needs Program

DISC Diagnostic Interview Schedule for Children

EPSDT Early and Periodic Screening, Diagnosis and Treatment

GAF Global Assessment of Functioning

HCFA Health Care Financing Administration
HEDIS Health Employer Data and Information Set
HIPAA Health Insurance Portability and Accountability Act
HMO Health maintenance organization

IPT Interpersonal psychotherapy

JCAHO Joint Commission on Accreditation of Healthcare Organizations

KSADS Kiddie Schedule for Affective Disorders and Schizophrenia

MCO Managed care organization
MHSIP Mental Health Statistics Improvement Program Consumer-Oriented Mental Health Report Card
MIS Management information system

NAMI   National Alliance for the Mentally Ill
NASMHPD   National Association of State Mental Health Program Directors
NCQA   National Committee for Quality Assurance
NIH   National Institutes of Health
NIMH   National Institute of Mental Health
NQF   National Quality Forum

ORYX   Not an acronym; refers to JCAHO's performance measurement program

PERMS   Performance measures
PMCC   Performance Measurement Coordinating Council
PORT   Patient Outcomes Research Team
PPG   Partnership Performance Grants (USDHHS set of behavioral health performance measures)

QA   Quality assurance
QAP   Quality assurance plan

SAMHSA   Substance Abuse and Mental Health Services Administration
S-CHIP   State Children's Health Insurance Program
SPMI   Severely and persistently mentally ill population

TIP   Treatment Improvement Protocol
TOPS   Treatment Outcome Prospective Study

USDHHS   U.S. Department of Health and Human Services

Glossary of Terms and Definitions

access   As used in the report, can refer to different facets of access. For example, does the service exist?; is it close by and convenient?; and, lastly, is it sufficiently available so health plan members can receive it as needed?

adolescent   Refers to an individual 13–18 years of age.

appropriate   As used in the report, refers to care, treatment, or interventions that are evidence-based or, in the absence of data, consistent with "best practices."

atypical antipsychotic   Refers to "novel" or "new generation" antipsychotic medications (i.e., risperidone, olanzapine, quetiapine, ziprasidone, and clozapine).

behavioral health care   Treatment for mental health problems, substance abuse, or both.

benefit package   What services a plan offers.

board certification   Designation given by the American Board of Psychiatry and Neurology (ABPN) for psychiatrists who have successfully completed the ABPN certification examination in *psychiatry* and child/adolescent psychiatrists who have successfully completed the additional ABPN certification examination in *child/adolescent psychiatry.* Child and adolescent psychiatrists must be ABPN certified in psychiatry before they can take the additional ABPN certification examination in child/adolescent psychiatry.

caregiver   See definition of family.

care management   Developing and authorizing the service plan and overseeing the coordination of care for a enrollee. Performed by an enrollee's individual service coordinator.

case management services   A process by which the services provided to a specific enrollee are managed to achieve optimum outcome in the most cost-effective manner.

child and adolescent psychiatrist   Licensed physician who has completed residency training in both general (adult) psychiatry and child/adolescent psychiatry.

child   Refers either broadly to any individuals less than 18 years of age or specifically to an individual less than 13 years of age.

Child and Adolescent Service System Program (CASSP)   Programs funded through a federal grant initiative that established new systems of care for children and adolescents with severe emotional disturbance.

comorbid or co-occurring condition   Refers to one or more psychiatric disorders or conditions that are present in addition to the primary diagnosis/disorder. For example, there is a significant number of children/adolescents with ADHD who also meet the diagnostic criteria for conduct disorder.

culturally appropriate   The capacity of individuals or organizations to effectively identify the health practices and behaviors of populations of concern; to design programs, interventions, and services that effectively address cultural and language barriers to the delivery of appropriate and necessary health care services; and to evaluate and contribute to the ongoing improvement of these efforts.

cultural assessment   Evaluation of language, customs, styles, values, beliefs, practices, groups, functions, processes, structure, procedures, and judgments of groups, organizations, or systems to ensure that no systemic barriers to appropriate service delivery exist.

cultural diversity   A constellation of people consisting of distinctive ethnic groups, colors and races, languages, customs, styles, values, beliefs, gender, ages, education, knowledge, skills, abilities, functions, practices, religions, and geographic areas.

cultural and linguistic competence   A set of congruent behaviors, attitudes, policies, and procedures that come together in a system, agency, or among professionals, enabling that system, agency, or those professionals to work effectively and efficiently in cross-cultural and diverse linguistic situations on a continuous basis. A culturally and linguistically competent system of care acknowledges and incorporates, at all levels, the importance of culture and language, the cultural strengths associated with people and communities, the assessment of cross-cultural relations, vigilance toward the dynamics inherent in cultural and linguistic differences, the expansion of cultural and linguistic knowledge, and the adaptation of services to meet culturally and linguistically unique needs.

cultural relevance   Services that bear "a traceable, significant, logical connection" to the culturally based needs, expectations, desires, and existential realities of the individuals to whom the services are directed; a leadership and work force that is able and willing to obtain the necessary knowledge about their clients' cultural and socioeconomic background that will enable them to plan and deliver effective therapeutic programs.

cultural sensitivity   Recognition and respect for customs and cultural norms different from one's own.

culture   Includes, but is not limited to, the shared values, norms, traditions, customs, arts, history, folklore, and religious and spiritual healing practices and institutions of a racial, ethnic, religious, or social group of people that are generally transmitted to succeeding generations.

diversity   The constellation and amalgamation of distinctive ethnic groups, colors, races, languages, customs, styles, values, beliefs, genders, education, knowledge, skills, abilities, functions, practices, and religions existing in a group, organization, or system.

DSM-IV   *Diagnostic and Statistical Manual of Mental Disorders,* 4th Edition, published by the American Psychiatric Association. It provides a complete classification of psychiatric disorders. A text revision of DSM-IV, referred to as DSM-IV-TR, appeared in 2000.

Early and Periodic Screening, Diagnosis and Treatment (EPSDT)   Medicaid entitlement program (Title XIX of the Social Security Act) for children and adolescents to age 21 that covers any medically necessary service allowable under Medicaid.

encounter   One visit or other transaction between a person and a plan provider.

episode of care   All the services provided for a specific condition over a continuous and specified period of time. Can be used to analyze cost of service, quality, and patterns of use.

ethnicity   A term that has been used loosely as a marker or statement of identity with a named grouping based on social (including own or ancestral history or geographic or national origin); linguistic, cultural, or biological characteristics; or political affiliation. Ethnic identifications may overlap, and an individual may identify him or herself, or be identified, with more than one named group with different boundaries in different social contexts. *Ethnicity* refers to membership in a group of people who share a unique social or cultural heritage that is passed on from generation to generation.

family   This word should be interpreted broadly to include parents or legal guardians, siblings, and other relatives living in the home and others with a significant role in child-rearing or the child's life. The concept of "a family" is diverse. Every family is unique and possesses its own culture, history, traditions, beliefs, strengths, and needs. What constitutes and functions as "a family" often transcends traditional definitions. Services developed and provided by a health plan should acknowledge and respect each individual family's uniqueness and diversity.

flexible services   See definition of wraparound services.

Global Assessment of Functioning (GAF) Scale   Single-item rating scale for evaluating overall psychosocial functioning during a specified time period on a continuum from psychological sickness to health.

Health Care Financing Administration (HCFA)   The federal agency with administrative responsibilities for Medicaid, Medicare, and child health insurance programs. The agency has been renamed Centers for Medicare and Medicaid Services (CMS).

health maintenance organization (HMO)   A health care organization that operates in a specific geographic area and offers comprehensive treatment and supplemental services to people who are enrolled. It is one type of managed care.

indicator (quality indicator)   A component of quality patient care.

indicated prevention   Refers to those interventions used with individuals who are at high risk for developing mental disorder in the future but who currently have minimal signs or symptoms (i.e., subclinical or subsyndromal) or have the prodromal phase of a disorder.

informed consent   Refers to the process of informing an individual who is providing consent (e.g., a parent for a child to take psychiatric medication) with all necessary and relevant information so they can make an "informed" choice/decision.

Joint Commission on the Accreditation of Healthcare Organizations (JCAHO)   A national organization dedicated to improving the quality of health care through accreditation services.

language   The medium of communication shared between a set of people. Language may be spoken or written and may also include gestures. *Dialect* is a distinct communication medium that can be traced historically to a language but which may not be mutually intelligible with other dialects related to the same language group or family. A native language provides a psychic bond or uniqueness that signifies membership in a particular ethnic group.

managed care   Various strategies that seek to maximize the value of services by controlling cost and use, promoting quality, and measuring performance to ensure cost-effectiveness.

managed care organization (MCO)   An organization that is responsible for evaluating enrollees' mental health needs; matching needs with appropriate resources; acquiring and managing the care (within the scope of a defined benefits package); paying for such care; coordinating mental health and substance abuse services with physical health care; and assuring the achievement of specific outcomes in the most cost-effective manner.

measure   A mechanism or instrument to quantify a quality indicator.

multicultural   Consisting of cultural characteristics representative of one or more ethnic groups. Multicultural individuals may acquire the norms, attitudes, and behavior patterns of their own and one or more other ethnic groups.

National Committee for Quality Assurance (NCQA)   An organization that evaluates and accredits medical services and quality management of managed care organizations.

network   A collection of providers assembled by a health maintenance organization or state-designated special needs plan to offer some or all required services.

outcomes   The impacts of a health plan on the individuals served and on the overall delivery system.

parent support services   Refers to a variety of services that provide parents of a child or adolescent with a mental disorder with support and assistance.

peer review   A quality assurance study of the appropriateness of how a clinician has provided services. It is conducted by people with comparable education and training.

performance indicators   Numerical summaries of performance obtained from instruments used to measure performance.

practice guidelines   Series of systematic "how-to's" of sound professional practice developed by the APA intended to guide treatment and improve the quality of services.

practice parameters   Series of systematic how-to's of sound professional practice developed by the AACAP intended to guide treatment and improve the quality of services.

practitioner   An individual who provides mental health services on a private fee-for-service basis or as an employee of a *provider* managed care organization or agency.

prevention-minded treatment   Refers to treatment interventions that are designed for those individuals with an identified mental illness who are at severe risk of progression of their mental illness, recurrence, relapse, or developing a co-occurring/comorbid mental disorder.

primary language   Primary language refers to the language an individual is most proficient in and uses most frequently to communicate with others inside and outside the family system. To provide equal access to individuals whose primary language is not English, mental health service providers offer mental health services through bilingual staff. When that is not possible, a qualified interpreter is provided at no cost to the client.

professional review organization   A group established by clinicians to review services for quality and appropriateness.

provider   An individual or organization that provides and is reimbursed for a health care service.

psychiatrist   Licensed physician who has completed residency training in general psychiatry.

qualified interpreter   A person who not only translates orally but also bridges the cultural gaps present in cross-cultural communication. Ideally, an interpreter should be someone who is trained in cross-cultural interpretation; trained in the health care field; proficient in the culture of the client and that of the health care professionals; and has an understanding of the significance of the particular health matter being discussed as well as an understanding of the importance of confidentiality.

quality assurance (QA)   A program or set of activities designed to monitor, evaluate, and improve care or services provided to enhance the health of enrollees and the effective use of resources, with an emphasis on improving health outcomes.

quality assurance plan (QAP)   Systematic plan to review and improve the quality of services provided.

race   Race is biologically defined as a semiclosed population exhibiting certain gene frequencies that may distinguish it from other populations. Because this is a biological definition, the term *race* when used in this way may have biomedical implications important to the provision of health services.

recommendation/goal   An important clinical principle that reflects quality patient care.

rehabilitation   Restoration of the highest practical functional level through education and therapy.

satisfaction/dissatisfaction   Subjective measurement of enrollee's and family members' evaluation of services related to access, appropriateness, outcomes, intrasystem/intersystem linkages, and prevention.

selected prevention   Refers to those interventions designed for use with individuals or a subgroup of a population who have a higher than average risk of developing a mental disorder.

serious emotional disturbance   A diagnosable mental disorder experienced by a child or adolescent that is sufficiently severe to cause significant impairment in functioning for at least 1 year, or significant impairment in functioning and severe symptoms for the previous 30 days.

services   The sum of those efforts, involving treatment, rehabilitation, and support, aimed at promoting mental health and reducing, eliminating, and otherwise ameliorating distress or disability caused by or associated with mental health problems, including services that may prevent reoccurrence of distress and/or dysfunction.

service planning   The ongoing delineation of goals, objectives, and therapeutic interventions and placement in the appropriate level of care based on the uniqueness of each individual client that incorporates the perspectives of the enrollee, the enrollee's clinician(s)/treatment team, family members, and/or significant others (only with permission of recipient). Treatment planning builds on the enrollee's abilities and incorporates a discharge focus.

stakeholders   People with a specific interest in seeing that a managed care plan runs appropriately. Examples of stakeholders are recipients of services, family members, service providers, state and local offices of mental health, and advocates.

standard   The level of a measure that suggests that the component of care is of adequate quality.

support   The application of resources to maintain an enrollee in the least restrictive environment, to encourage an enrollee to fully reach identified health goals, and to assist the enrollee in achieving desired outcomes.

translation   Putting words of one language into another, particularly in written form. In health services, translation is used when converting written information from English-language medical/psychiatric forms, information brochures, and other health-related materials into the enrollee's primary language. Translation involves a review of materials for cultural and linguistic appropriateness.

universal prevention   Refers to those interventions that would benefit everyone in the general population or a population subgroup. These interventions are targeted to the general population or a whole population of a specific group but not identified on the basis of individual risk.

utilization management   A system of procedures designed to ensure that the services provided to a specific enrollee at a given time are cost-effective, appropriate, and least restrictive.

utilization review   An analysis of services used to determine how costs can be contained or reduced and effectiveness increased.

wraparound services   An essential component of individualized, community-based care for children and adolescents with severe emotional disturbance. These services are unconditional, flexible, and child/family-focused. The services follow or wraparound the child or adolescent to facilitate return to optimal functioning at home and in the community. Examples are after-school programs, summer camp, recreation programs, mentoring, life coaches, parent aides, and community supervision.

Index of Quality Indicators by Topic

Note: This index contains an **alphabetical listing by topic** of all the sample quality indicators contained in this report. In addition, there are two subset listings of indicators organized by psychiatric disorders and treatment interventions.

The quality indicators contained in the report were selected as *representative samples* for each domain. This report is not intended to be a comprehensive compilation of all possible quality indicators in child and adolescent mental health.

Topics (alphabetical) *(continued)*

Disorders Subset

Topics (alphabetical)	Quality indicator	Page
ADHD (attention-deficit/hyperactivity disorder)	C.2b.1.1	108
	B.3a.1.1	97
	B.3b.1.1	98
	E.2.1.1	129
Anxiety disorder	C.2a.1.1	106
Conduct disorder	B.3a.1.1	97
Depression	A.4.1.1	91
	B.3b.1.1	98
	C.2a.1.1	106
Obsessive-compulsive disorder (OCD)	B.3b.1.2	98
	C.2a.1.1	106
Oppositional defiant disorder (ODD)	B.3a.1.1	97
Psychosis	C.2b.1.2	109
	E.3.1.3	134
Speech and language services/disorders	B.3c.1.1	99
Substance abuse treatment/disorder	D.1a.1.1	117
	E.2.1.1	129
	E.2.1.2	130
Subsyndromal symptoms of depression, anxiety, and eating disorders	A.3.1.1	89

Interventions Subset

Interventions (alphabetical)	Quality indicator	Page
Behavior management	B.3a.1.1	97
Cognitive-behavioral therapy (CBT)	C.2a.1.1	106
Interpersonal psychotherapy (IPT)	C.2a.1.2	107
Medications		
Anti-OCD	B.3b.1.2	98
Atypical antipsychotics	C.2b.1.2	109
SSRIs	B.3b.1.3	98
Stimulants	C.2b.1.1	108
	B.3b.1.1	98
Parent skills building	A.2.2.1	85
Psychoeducation	A.4.1.1	91
Speech and language services/disorders	B.3c.1.1	99
Substance abuse treatment/disorder	D.1a.1.1	117
	E.2.1.1	129
	E.2.1.2	130

Index of Surveys, Rating Scales, and Instruments

Measure	Quality indicator	Page
Diagnostic instruments		
K-SADS (Schedule for Affective Disorders and Schizophrenia for School-Age Children)	C.1.1.1	105
NIMH-DISC (Diagnostic Interview Schedule for Children)	C.1.1.1	105
Functional assessment instruments		
CAFAS (Child and Adolescent Functional Assessment Scale)	E.3.1.3	134
CANS (Child and Adolescent Needs and Strengths)	E.3.1.3	134
CHQ (Child Health Questionnaire)	E.4.1.1	135
PPQ-A (Patient Problem Questionnaire for Adolescents)	A.1.1.1	82
Family functioning instruments		
CAIA (Child and Adolescent Impact Assessment)	E.5.1.1	137
Caregiver Strain Questionnaire	E.5.1.1	137
Satisfaction surveys/instruments		
CABHS (Consumer Assessment of Behavioral Health Services)	D.1a.1.1	117
	D.1b.1.1	118
	D.1c.1.1	119
	D.2a.1.1	120
	D.2c.1.1	122
CCCI-R (Cross Cultural Counseling Inventory)	D.1b.1.1	118
	D.1c.1.1	119
	D.2b.1.1	121
FACS (Parent Assessment of Care Survey)	D.2a.1.1	120
	D.2b.1.1	121
	D.2c.1.1	122
Tools for Monitoring Cultural Competence	D.1b.1.1	118
	D.1c.1.1	119
	D.2b.1.1	121
Restrictiveness of placements		
ROLES (Restrictiveness of Living Environments Scale)	E.7.1.1	141

Index to Report of the APA Task Force on Quality Indicators

Index to Report of the APA Task Force on Quality Indicators for Children